2006
Men'sHealth®
TOTAL
FITNESS
GUIDE

RODALE®

© 2006 by Rodale Inc.

All rights reserved. No part of this publication may be reproduced or transmitted in any form or by any means, electronic or mechanical, including photocopying, recording, or any other information storage and retrieval system, without the written permission of the publisher.

Men's Health is a registered trademark of Rodale Inc.

Printed in the United States of America
Rodale Inc. makes every effort to use acid-free ∞, recycled paper ♺.

2   4   6   8   10   9   7   5   3   1   hardcover

Visit us on the Web at www.menshealthbooks.com, or call us toll-free at (800) 848-4735.

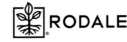

RODALE®

WE **INSPIRE** AND **ENABLE** PEOPLE TO IMPROVE
THEIR LIVES AND THE WORLD AROUND THEM

2006 Men'sHealth TOTAL FITNESS GUIDE

EDITOR-IN-CHIEF, *MEN'S HEALTH* MAGAZINE
David Zinczenko

EXECUTIVE EDITOR
Zachary Schisgal

EDITOR
Deanna Portz

EXERCISE ADVISOR
Michael Mejia, CSCS

CONTRIBUTING WRITERS
Adam Bean; Mike Clark, MS, PT; Kate Dailey; Matt Fitzgerald; Jeff Galloway; Liesa Goins; Timothy Gower; Ben Hewitt; Noah Liberman; Michael Mejia, CSCS; Brian Metzler; Peter Moore; Myatt Murphy; Stephen Perrine; Scott Quill; Phillip Rhodes; Lara Rosenbaum; David Schipper; Lou Schuler; Heidi Skolnik, MS, CDN; Ian Smith, MD; Ted Spiker; D. Milton Stokes, RD; Trevor Thieme; Mark Verstegen, MS, CSCS; Alison Wellner; John R. White Jr., PharmD; Allison Winn Scotch; Mike Zimmerman

INTERIOR DESIGNER
Sandy Freeman

COVER DESIGNER
Christopher Rhoads

PHOTO EDITOR
Darleen Malkames

ASSOCIATE PHOTO EDITOR
Robin Hepler

COPY EDITOR
Rachelle Vander Schaaf

PROJECT MANAGER
Lois Hazel

LAYOUT DESIGNER
Keith Biery

PRODUCT SPECIALIST
Jodi Schaffer

SENIOR MANAGING EDITOR
Chris Krogermeier

SENIOR MANAGER, MULTIMEDIA PRODUCTION SERVICES
Robert V. Anderson Jr.

PAGE ASSEMBLY MANAGER
Patricia Brown

VICE PRESIDENT, ART AND DESIGN
Andy Carpenter

MANAGING ART DIRECTOR
Darlene Schneck

PRESIDENT, EDITOR-IN-CHIEF
Tami Booth Corwin

SENIOR VICE PRESIDENT, PUBLISHER, DIRECT RESPONSE BOOKS
Gregg Michaelson

SENIOR DIRECTOR, DIRECT RESPONSE MARKETING
Janine Slaughter

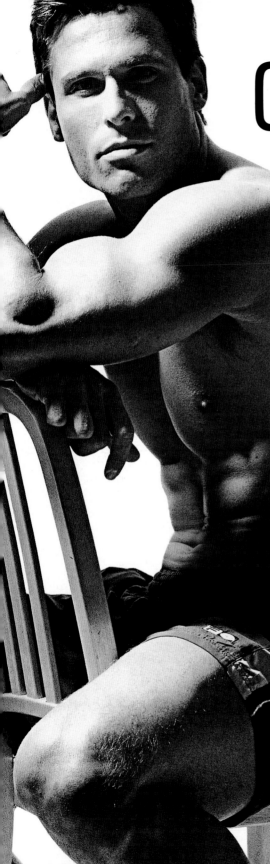

Contents

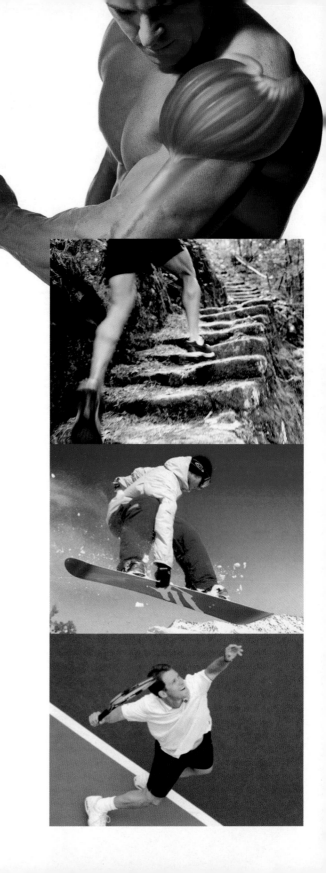

Introduction

The Latest and Greatest

As the sports and nutrition editor of *Men's Health*, I'm frequently asked by our readers how we manage—month after month and year after year—to create fresh stories on the "same old topics." The short answer, of course, is that it's not easy.

But beyond sharing tales of staff creativity and resourcefulness, I must confess that we'll never have to worry about a shortage of new and useful material to fill our pages. That's because the fitness and nutrition industry is constantly evolving, in much the same way as the medical field.

Think about it: You'd never assume that we've seen the end of advancements in medicine. In fact, you *expect* to see new therapies, procedures, and medications developed on a regular basis. So why should you presume that you've seen your last cutting-edge training method, diet improvement, or weight-loss shortcut? The truth is, you haven't. In fact, the best is yet to come.

Case in point: the information on the pages of this book. Whether your goal is to build muscle, lose fat, or—if you're like most guys—do both, you'll find innovative but practical tips that you can start putting to use today, both in the kitchen and the weight room, as well as on the treadmill. If you prefer to shape up outside, you'll relish the tips starting on page 178 that are especially for guys hitting the slopes, court, and trail. For a comprehensive exercise-by-exercise, set-by-set, how-to plan, check out "Make Your Workout Work Harder for You" on page 43 by *Men's Health* exercise advisor and world-class strength coach Michael Mejia, CSCS. It's designed to help you achieve the best results in the time you have—even if you can spare only 2 days a week. And if it's motivation you need, we provide that, too—21 new ways to eliminate the most common excuses for skipping a workout.

You see, the problems—lack of know-how, time, and inspiration—never change. But the solutions do. And you now hold the proof in your hands. Think you can't improve your workout and diet? The *2006 Men's Health Total Fitness Guide* is guaranteed to make you think again.

—ADAM CAMPBELL

MANAGE YOUR
WAIST

At *Men's Health*, we make it our job to give you the knowledge and tools to help you be a winner at everything you do, from building a better body and beating stress to advancing in your career. So it may come as a surprise to find out we want to help you become a big loser.

We're referring to you losing that gut of yours—once and for all. In our all-you-can-eat society, with Golden Arches and greasy spoons at every street corner, it's no wonder so many of us are lugging around a spare tire. If you're ready to off-load yours, you've come to the right place. We've done the research, talked to weight-loss experts, and pored over recipe books—so you don't have to. In the pages that follow, we reveal diets that work, make ordering out easier, and offer solutions to seven of the most common dieting roadblocks. We make losing weight so easy, the pounds are sure to drop in no time.

The only thing we *don't* provide are smaller pants. You're gonna have to spring for those yourself, you big loser.

BY ALLISON WINN SCOTCH

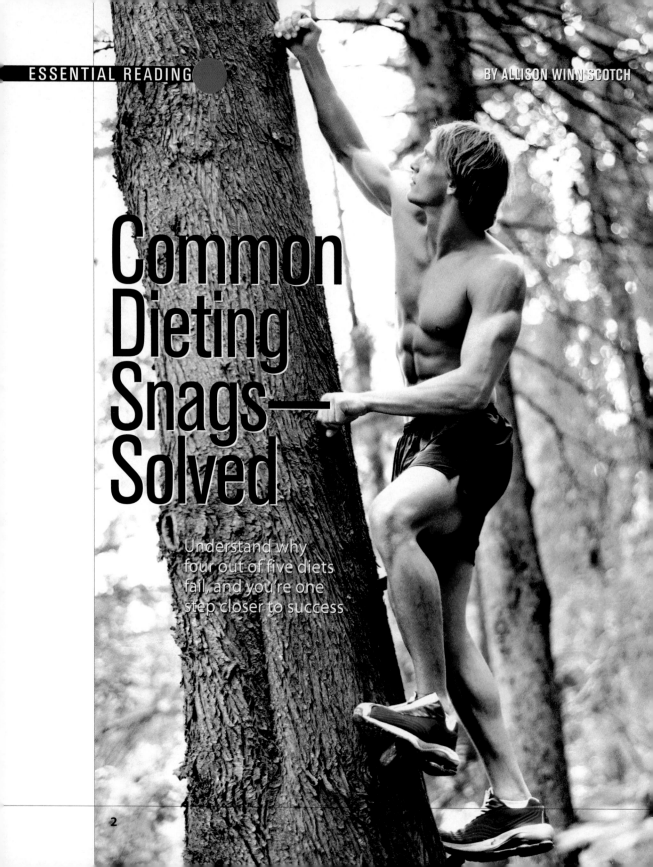

Common Dieting Snags— Solved

Understand why four out of five diets fail, and you're one step closer to success

Dieting sucks. The deprivation, the siren calls of beer and pizza, the annoyance of micromanagement. Worst of all is the sense that the diet will last forever, that the peppery tang of chicken wings will never again touch your lips. It's no surprise that 80 percent of diets go belly-up, according to the *American Journal of Clinical Nutrition.*

We won't tell you to skip the diet altogether. We will tell you that it's going to be okay, though. In order to prevail, you simply have to get inside the diet's whens, hows, and whys.

So this time, instead of stumbling blindly through treacherous territory, you're going to go on a guided tour of potential diet pitfalls—maybe the same ones that have snared you before. And this time, you'll breeze past them.

There's just one catch: A new you is just a few months away. Ready to meet him?

1 Week

The crisis: You're freakin' starving.

Before: You ate the first thing you saw.

Now: Eat, but eat differently. Grab foods with lots of fiber and water. Your (gut) instinct says you want a Burger King Whopper with Cheese. Your smarter self knows that the same caloric load is found in a bowl of whole-wheat pasta with tomatoes and spinach, a whole-wheat dinner roll, a bowl of soup, and three scoops of sorbet. In the car? You'll keep a stash of dried fruit—a tasty, nutrient-rich hunger-killer.

The science: When your stomach is empty, the hormone ghrelin kicks in, which stimulates appetite, says Scott Isaacs, MD, a clinical instructor of medicine at Emory University in Atlanta and author of *Hormonal Balance.* Don't let that happen. "By eating foods that are packed with fiber and water, such as fruits and vegetables, you'll feel full while controlling ghrelin production," he says. Protein does the same thing, but some protein-rich foods are calorie-rich, too. So alternate. Have high-protein string cheese in the morning, fiber- and water-rich apple slices in the afternoon.

The crisis: You're cranky.

Before: You grabbed chips and a soda.

Now: Boost your mood with snacks that satisfy your hormones, not your stomach. Fatty, sugary foods quickly turn into glucose after digestion. From now on, your snacks will be complex carbohydrates, such as a whole-grain treat like a bowl of Cheerios with blueberries and 2 percent milk.

The science: You're cranky because you've eliminated sources of quick mood-boosting energy—like chips and colas. "When these easy sources of energy are cut, you're going to go through a time when you don't feel great," says Vincent Pera, MD, director of the weight-management program at Miriam Hospital in Providence, Rhode Island. Researchers in the Netherlands recently demonstrated that a glucose infusion can help ward off feelings of anxiety by enhancing serotonin function. That's fine, but get your boost from complex carbohydrates that raise your serotonin levels without inflating your waistline the way sugary carbs can.

1 Month

The crisis: The scale seems stuck.

Before: You figured, *What's the point? This isn't working.*

Now: Get in gear. "Exercising is critical at this juncture," says Dr. Isaacs. Nothing complicated—just move. Cardiovascular exercise (running, biking, hoops) burns calories, and lifting weights increases muscle mass, which will make you burn more calories even while you're sleeping. For each pound of muscle you add, you burn an extra 20 to 50 calories a day. And drink lots of water to replace what you're sweating out. Staying hydrated helps your body break down fat and deadens those hunger pangs. (After all, water takes up stomach space, too.)

The science: "As you lose weight, you require fewer calories, but by building muscle mass, you'll rev up your metabolism and counter this effect," Dr. Isaacs says. In a recent study at the University of Arkansas, people on low-fat, high-complex-carbohydrate diets who also exercised lost 3.5 pounds more over 12 weeks than those who ate similar diets but skipped the gym.

Prescription Pitfalls

Three common medicines that can mess with your weight

DRUG	FAT FACTOR	STRATEGY
Imitrex (sumatriptan) For severe migraines	Fluid retention	Try older medications, like Endolor.
Prednisone (corticosteroids, glucocorticoids) Anti-inflammatory	Sodium retention, leading to extra water weight	Try a different drug in the same class, like methylprednisolone.
Propecia (finasteride) For baldness and enlarged prostate	Enlarged breasts from water retention	For baldness, try an OTC minoxidil treatment. If you're taking Propecia for your prostate, ask about alpha-blockers, which relax smooth muscles in the bladder and prostate.

Source: Christopher Forst, RPh, MPA, FAPhA, director of pharmacy at Health South Medical Center in Dallas

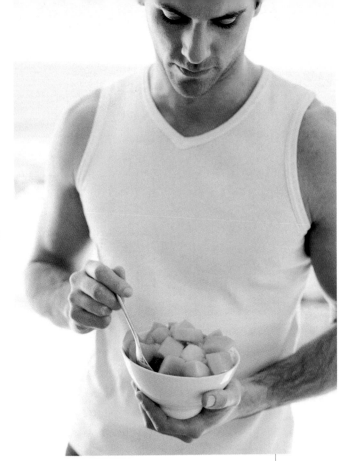

The crisis: You have intense food cravings.

Before: You gave in. Because, hey, life is meant to be enjoyed.

Now: Give in to snack attacks, but wisely. David Katz, MD, director of the prevention research center at Yale University School of Medicine and author of *The Way to Eat*, recommends carrying "the food equivalent of an umbrella." Keep a bag or small cooler of nuts, fruits, yogurt, and low-fat cheese on hand at all times. You need ready access to healthy sources of protein or fiber to offset sudden, out-of-nowhere cravings.

The science: "When you diet, your previously overstuffed fat cells start shrinking," Dr. Katz says. They know their number's up and that they'll soon be burned for fuel. Understandably, they have other plans. "These cells send a message to your brain saying that they need more fuel. They shut down production of leptin, the hormone that tells your brain you're satisfied," he says. So your brain, by way of your cells, goes on the hunt for anything it can get your hands on—which is why you should keep healthy snacks within easy reach.

6 Months

The crisis: You've made so much progress that you think, *What the hell.*

Before: You slipped—face-first, into a double-pepperoni, extra-cheese pizza.

Now: Weigh in. You need to keep your eye on your rate of weight loss. Setting targets blows away complacency. "People taste success, and their adherence slips," Dr. Pera says. "Their initial feelings of urgency to lose the weight also diminish."

The science: A study at the University of Massachusetts at Dartmouth shows that people who weigh themselves regularly are more likely to stay focused. They're continually reminded of their success so far and of the road ahead. Reaching your goal weight makes you more likely to keep the pounds off. A researcher at the University of Pennsylvania reports that patients who achieve their weight-loss goals are more psychologically satisfied. You're likely to stick with anything—a job, tennis practice—when you know it's paying off.

The crisis: You reach a plateau.

Before: You figure, *Well, that's it. I've come far enough.*

Now: Diet less, exercise more. It's probably going to be easier to exercise more frequently than to further restrict a diet that's become an ingrained habit. Throw in a few high-intensity days—an extralong run or bike ride—to boost the calorie deficit. If your exercise is mostly cardiovascular, devote more time to weight lifting.

The science: "Because your caloric needs have lessened, you need to burn off more in order to continue to see results," Dr. Pera says. "If you don't increase your amount of exercise or continue to cut calories, you plateau." The muscle from weight lifting, Dr. Katz says, will "increase resting energy expenditure. Then, when you return to more aerobics, you're taking more calorie-burning muscle with you, and you'll be bumped off the plateau."

9 Months

The crisis: A voice in your head says, *I want my life back.*

Before: You got fat again.

Now: Let loose—a little bit. "Being on a strict diet can drain you mentally, so there's a huge temptation to let things slide," says Dr. Katz. If you're meeting your goals, give yourself a break. "If you love ice cream, try a lower-fat version or a sorbet," suggests Howard M. Shapiro, MD, author of *Dr.*

Shapiro's Picture Perfect Weight Loss. "A pint of Ben & Jerry's Phish Food ice cream has 1,200 calories, while a pint of sorbet has only 300. You can still enjoy the taste, but you're not inflicting so much damage." The same logic applies with pizza, cake, beer—you name it. Savor a cold one, but make it an Amstel Light. Instead of the all-meat, extra-cheese pizza, top yours with chicken and green peppers.

The science: "By making your choices, you are empowered and in control and won't feel the deprivation that might lead you to quit," Dr. Shapiro says. When you feel as if you've cultivated enough willpower, reintroduce a couple of all-time favorites into your diet—as treats, not everyday fare. If you've made it this far, you deserve a Guinness and an order of chicken wings—the baked ones, thanks.

1 Year

The crisis: There is none.

Now: "Physiologically, you've converted your body from a foe to an ally," says Dr. Katz. Blur the line between diet and lifestyle. Now that healthier eating patterns are ingrained, your diet isn't a "diet" any longer—it's a new way of living.

The science: According to research by the North American Association for the Study of Obesity, successful dieters report that "significantly less" effort is required to maintain weight loss; as the pounds come off, less conscious attention is needed to keep them off. In other words, the longer you go, the easier it gets.

BY D. MILTON STOKES, RD

Eat More, Weigh Less

Scarfing six meals a day boosts energy, builds muscle, and sheds pounds. But what to eat? Here's your quick 'n' easy guide

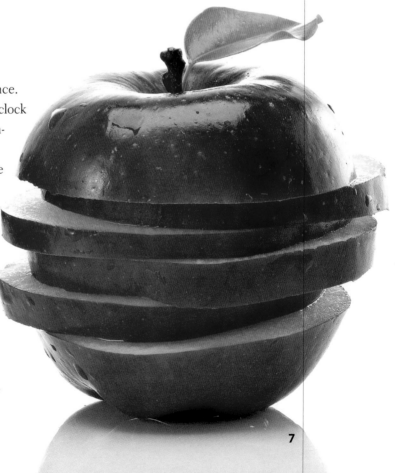

S ome things are sadly predictable. Extra winter poundage, for instance. Or holiday binges. Or the three o'clock slump, which sags before you like a hammock every afternoon.

Here's a happier prediction: Eat more often and you'll avoid all of those problems. Spreading six smaller meals across your day operates on the simple principle of satisfaction. Frequent meals tame the slavering beast of hunger. The secret? Each mini meal should blend protein and fiber-rich complex carbohydrates. "Protein and fiber give you that feeling of satiety and keep you from feeling hungry," says Tara Geise, RD, a nutritionist in private practice in Orlando and a spokeswoman

7

for the American Dietetic Association (ADA).

Controlling hunger shrinks your gut. In a study published in the *International Journal of Obesity,* one group of overweight men was given five small meals, then was free to choose a sixth meal. A second group ate a single meal containing the same number of calories as the total of the other group's first five meals, then later had a free-choice second meal. The six-meal men ate 27 percent less food at their last meal than the two-meal men did at their second.

Consistent eating will also keep your protein levels high, helping you build muscle. "Your body can metabolize only so much protein at one time," says Katherine Tallmadge, RD, author of *Diet Simple.* "Protein is metabolized better when it's divided evenly."

The challenge is keeping the mini meals mini. "It's critical that at the end of the day, the calorie content of your mini meals does not exceed what you would eat in three larger meals," says Jeannie Moloo, PhD, RD, an ADA spokeswoman in Roseville, California.

If you already know your calorie count, start eating. Otherwise, go to www.Mens Health.com/caloriecalc and plug in your weight and activity level. With a suggested calorie count in hand, you can mix and match from the list of meals shown here. Yes, you can take two items from one meal list—if they're small. Looking to lose? Choose lower-calorie options. Regular Joe? Be as flexible as you please. Building muscle? Double up on a couple of the items—have an extra slice of pizza or two containers of yogurt.

Breakfast (6 to 8:30 A.M.)

You're sleepy, so we'll keep it simple: Mix protein and quality carbs. "When protein is included in a meal, not only does it help prevent overeating at other times of day, but it also sustains energy levels and improves concentration," says Bonnie Taub-Dix, MA, RD, CDN, an ADA spokeswoman. This means choosing a milk-infused latte instead of plain coffee, or a slather of peanut butter along with the jelly on an English muffin. Do not leave home without breakfast—this is the foundation for the rest of your day.

110 calories: Latte with reduced-fat milk

140 calories: Skippy brand Squeeze Stix peanut butter snack

200 calories: 1 cup reduced-sodium cottage cheese with fresh peaches and cinnamon

200 calories: 1 cup blackberries, blueberries, or strawberries with 6 ounces light yogurt and 1 tablespoon low-fat granola

250 calories: Any-way-you-like-it egg on a whole-grain English muffin with melted cheese

250 calories: Oatmeal made with reduced-fat milk instead of water; add brown sugar, walnuts, and/or any fresh or dried fruit

260 calories: Cold whole-grain cereal, such as Kashi or raisin bran, with reduced-fat milk

300 calories: Peanut butter and jelly on a whole-grain English muffin

300 calories: Scrambled-egg burrito with turkey sausage and salsa

300 calories: 2-egg omelet with spinach, mushrooms, and feta cheese

Midmorning Snack (9:30 to 10:30 A.M.)

Planning matters. If there's nothing but junk in your workplace vending machines, buy the foods you need—string cheese, granola bars, trail mix, whatever—and keep a stash at your desk. (See "Make It, Take It" below.)

80 calories: Stick of string cheese

100 calories: Hard-boiled egg with a handful of grape tomatoes

180 calories: Nature Valley granola bar

250 calories: Ready-made reduced-fat smoothie, such as Stonyfield Farm

250 calories: Clif bar

275 calories: 2 or 3 small handfuls of trail mix

290 calories: Kellogg's Nutri-Grain bar with a handful of pistachios or almonds

300 calories: Slice of whole-grain bread topped with peanut butter and banana

Make It, Take It
Because a bag lunch doesn't have to be boring

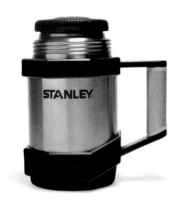

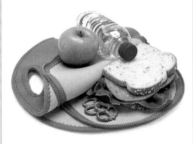

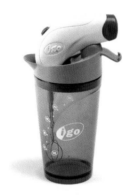

Stanley Bolt Food Jar

Keep it hot. This widemouthed industrial riff on the classic Stanley thermos is vacuum-insulated. Grab the handle, lift, and chug. Octagonal end caps make it roll-proof to keep it from becoming a soup-filled projectile during the morning commute. ($20; www.stanley-pmi.com)

Built NY BYO Lunch Bag

Hold it steady. If neoprene kept Jacques Cousteau cozy below the sea, this wet-suit-wannabe bag should do just fine with your lunch. With drink and meal pockets, the bag un-zips to form a place mat, in case you're handcuffed to your desk. ($26; www.builtny.com)

Igo Mix & Go Mini Mixer

Mix it up. This no-nonsense mini mixer nests in a 16-ounce cup that fits in a cup holder or desk drawer. Measuring marks mean you can skip the scoops, and the splash-resistant lid keeps your lapels spill-free, even when you're mixing up the sloppiest of protein shakes. ($20; www.igohomeproducts.com)

300 calories: Small bagel with 2 slices of Muenster cheese, melted

400 calories: Medium-size fruit muffin (best if made with whole-wheat flour)

Lunch (12 to 1:30 P.M.)

Be careful here! If you've had only a latte, fruit, and some string cheese so far, go ahead and have a big lunch. But if you've already eaten 700 calories (an omelet and a muffin, say), keep lunch light. Whatever you do, eat slowly, no matter how un-American that seems. It'll help you feel satisfied—and keep you that way.

175 calories: Canned tuna with balsamic vinegar on whole-grain crackers or bread

300 calories: 3 corn-tortilla flautas stuffed with refried beans and dipped in salsa

350 calories: Half an avocado, sliced, or ½ cup prepared guacamole with tomato and onion in a whole-grain pita

375 calories: Baked potato with chopped broccoli and a slice of American cheese, melted

400 calories: Seafood salad in a whole-grain pita with diced tomato, cucumber, and onion

400 calories: 3 or 4 slices of bacon, reduced-fat Cheddar cheese, thin apple slices, and peanut butter on toasted whole-grain bread

400 calories: ½ cup hummus with roasted vegetables

400 calories: Small ham-, turkey-, or roast-beef-and-Swiss wrap with vegetables and mustard in a whole-wheat tortilla

400 calories: Fresh mozzarella and

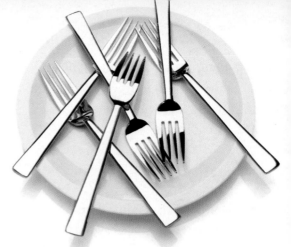

tomato slices on a bed of greens, with balsamic vinaigrette and extra-virgin olive oil

450 calories: 6 pierogi with salsa or reduced-fat sour cream

Midafternoon Snack (2:30 to 3:30 P.M.)

Steer clear of the candy bowl on your office manager's desk. "You could eat four small chocolates for 100 calories," says Geise, "or you could eat a cup of yogurt." The chocolate gives you hardly any protein; the yogurt delivers 8 grams.

160 calories: Reduced-fat Cheddar melted on apple halves

175 calories: 5 Laughing Cow cheese wedges

200 calories: ½ cup baba ghannouj (roasted-eggplant dip) with vegetables

210 calories: Half a container of Cracker Jack

250 calories: 1 cup reduced-fat yogurt

250 calories: Small handful of chopped pecans over a cup of fruit salad

260 calories: Apple, pear, or banana smeared with peanut butter

300 calories: Cup of chickpeas with a dash of cumin and fresh mint

340 calories: 2 ounces roasted nuts

350 calories: 1 cup each fat-free milk and frozen yogurt blended with a spoonful of peanut butter

Dinner (5:30 to 7:30 P.M.)

Okay, this isn't dinner as you used to know it. But don't panic. At first, reining in meal sizes will seem strange. But portion control can make or break the plan. "This is crucial, whether you're looking to control weight, manage blood sugar, or maintain energy levels," says Tallmadge. And remember—you'll be eating again in 2 hours.

200 calories: 2 cups mixed vegetables (fresh or frozen) with ½ cup marinara sauce and some grated Parmesan cheese

275 calories: 3 or 4 large handfuls of greens sautéed in olive oil with a handful of walnuts and ½ cup raisins

300 calories: 6-piece sushi meal with a cup of miso soup

325 calories: Buffalo burger topped with coleslaw, onion, and tomato

350 calories: Quesadilla made with a small corn or whole-wheat tortilla, cheese, beans, shredded chicken or lean ground beef, onion, and jalapeños, and dipped in salsa

400 calories: Slice of pizza topped with cheese and ground beef or ham

400 calories: Turkey London broil cut into strips and sautéed with onion, red and orange bell pepper, and teriyaki sauce

450 calories: Small plateful of nachos—baked tortilla chips, shredded reduced-fat cheese, refried beans, and salsa (plus some corn or black beans, if you want)

500 calories: Lentil, minestrone, or tomato soup with a grilled cheese sandwich on whole-grain bread

550 calories: 1 cup pasta tossed with browned ground turkey breast, black olives, diced onion, a drizzle of olive oil, and 1½ tablespoons crumbled Gorgonzola cheese

Evening Snack (8:30 to 10 P.M.)

Famished? Feeling as if this was the longest day of your life? Maybe your calorie count is too low. Adjust it by adding more sensible foods to your plan. Or choose higher-fiber foods; they're digested slowly, so they'll help you feel fuller longer.

150 calories: 5 cups Jolly Time light microwave popcorn sprinkled with hot sauce and/or 1 tablespoon of Romano cheese

150 calories: 1 cup rice pudding

150 calories: 6 or 7 strawberries dipped in yogurt and drizzled with chocolate sauce

150 calories: 1 cup cocoa made with fat-free milk

175 calories: Sliced sweet potato (with skin), tossed in olive oil and baked

175 calories: 1 cup fat-free ricotta cheese sweetened with Splenda, vanilla flavoring, and a dash of nutmeg or cinnamon

175 calories: Seltzer with 2 scoops frozen yogurt, a handful of berries, and a shot of flavoring syrup, such as strawberry or cherry

200 calories: Root-beer float with 2 scoops of frozen vanilla yogurt

200 calories: 2 handfuls of olives

275 calories: 2-ounce Snickers bar

BY PHILLIP RHODES

50 Ways to Feed Your Muscles

The skinless chicken breast is one of the leanest, most protein-packed foods you can eat. It's also boring. Here's how to keep it delicious, meal after meal

Every family argues about what to eat for dinner. But the Shrader family of Bluebell, West Virginia, took dinner-table combat to a whole new level one summer evening two years ago when 49-year-old Jackie Lee and his son, Harley Lee, 24, whipped out .22-caliber pistols and exchanged fire after sparring over how to cook their meal.

What food could trigger a kitchen gun battle? The harmless, boneless, skinless—and often flavorless—chicken breast, that's what. Sure, this omnipresent cut of poultry is the leanest source of protein this side of tofu or fish—a single serving offers 26 grams of protein for the price of 1 gram of saturated fat. But it's boring as hell.

And it doesn't help that most people eat their annual average of 88 pounds one of two ways: soaked in Italian salad dressing or slathered in barbecue sauce.

In my mind, that's exactly how I hear the Shrader feud erupting. "Marinade!" one might have said. "No! Barbecue sauce," the other yelled. Back and forth it went until it came to blows, then bullets. (Harley Lee took a slug to the head but managed to survive.) That's why I came up with this list—not one, not two, but 50 different ways to prepare a chicken breast. What good is eating healthy food if the boredom nearly kills you?

Stir-Frying

Basic technique: Cut the raw chicken into bite-size pieces or thin strips. Cook them in a nonstick skillet or wok over medium-high heat for 3 to 5 minutes or until browned. Then add the remaining ingredients from one of our stir-fry options in the order listed. Cook for 5 more minutes, stirring frequently. *Tip:* Sesame oil gives stir-fries their distinct flavor. Like olive oil, it's high in the unsaturated fats you want but olive oil can burn at high temperatures. Or, you can use canola or peanut oil.

1. 1 Tbsp reduced-sodium soy sauce; 2 tsp sesame oil; $\frac{1}{2}$ c green or red bell pepper, cut into strips; $\frac{1}{4}$ medium onion, cut lengthwise into strips; $\frac{1}{2}$ tsp red pepper flakes

2. 1 Tbsp hoisin sauce; 2 tsp sesame oil; $\frac{1}{3}$ c matchstick carrots; $\frac{1}{3}$ c chopped celery; 1 green onion, sliced; 2 Tbsp chopped, unsalted peanuts

3. 1 Tbsp reduced-sodium soy sauce; 2 tsp sesame oil; $\frac{1}{2}$ c asparagus tips; 2 Tbsp chopped, unsalted cashews

4. 1 Tbsp reduced-sodium soy sauce; 1 Tbsp lemon juice; 1 tsp lemon zest; 1 tsp honey; 1 clove garlic, crushed; $\frac{1}{2}$ c snow peas; 1 c chopped celery

5. 1 whisked egg; $\frac{1}{2}$ c (or more) chopped broccoli; $\frac{1}{4}$ medium onion, cut lengthwise into strips; $\frac{1}{2}$ tsp red pepper flakes; 1 Tbsp reduced-sodium soy sauce

6. 1 whisked egg; $\frac{1}{2}$ c snow peas; $\frac{1}{2}$ c green or red bell pepper, cut into strips; $\frac{1}{4}$ onion, cut lengthwise into strips; 1 Tbsp hoisin sauce

Baking

Basic technique: Preheat the oven to 350°F while you sauce, rub, crust, or stuff your chicken breast using any one of the recipes on the following pages. Then, bake the chicken breast for 20 to 25 minutes, or until an internal roasting thermometer reaches 170°. Don't overcook it. Err on the side of tenderness. An overcooked, dried-out chicken breast won't give you salmonella, but you probably won't want to eat it in the first place. *Tip:* Quickly searing the breast in a hot skillet will help avoid dryness because it locks in the bird's juices.

SAUCED

Watery ready-made sauces like salsa will bake fine—some of the liquid boils away as the chicken bakes. But thicker sauces, like barbecue or ranch, need water or broth mixed in; otherwise you'll be left with a sticky, blackened char. *Tip:* Use a small baking dish to keep the meat covered with sauce.

7. $1/3$ c salsa

8. 2 Tbsp jalapeño cheese dip, 2 Tbsp salsa, 1 Tbsp water

9. 2 Tbsp marinara sauce, 2 Tbsp water

10. 2 Tbsp barbecue sauce, 2 Tbsp water

11. 2 Tbsp ranch dressing, 2 Tbsp water

12. 2 Tbsp Dijon mustard, 2 Tbsp honey, 1 tsp olive oil

13. 3 Tbsp chicken broth; 1 Tbsp mustard; 1 clove garlic, crushed

14. 2 Tbsp condensed cream of mushroom soup, 2 Tbsp water

15. 2 Tbsp pesto, 2 Tbsp reduced-sodium chicken broth

16. 2 Tbsp reduced-sodium soy sauce, $1/4$ c crushed pineapple with juice

17. 3 Tbsp chicken broth, 2 Tbsp light coconut milk, $1/4$ tsp curry powder

18. $1/3$ c chicken broth, 1 Tbsp maple syrup, 1 Tbsp apple juice

19. 3 Tbsp red wine vinegar; 1 Tbsp barbecue sauce; 1 clove garlic, crushed

20. 2 Tbsp hot sauce, 2 Tbsp Worcestershire sauce, $1/4$ tsp chili powder

21. 2 Tbsp lemon juice, 2 Tbsp orange marmalade, $1/4$ tsp rosemary

RUBBED

Rub one of the following spice mixtures evenly over each breast, then hit the chicken with a shot or two of cooking spray (not too much, though) to hold the rub in place and help form a light crust when cooking.

22. **Tex-Mex style:** $1/4$ tsp each garlic powder, chili powder, black pepper, and oregano; pinch of salt

23. **Southwestern:** $1/4$ tsp each black pepper, chili powder, red pepper flakes, cumin, and hot sauce

24. **French:** $1/4$ tsp each dried basil, rosemary, and thyme; pinch of salt and pepper

CRUSTED

A whisked egg acts like glue, holding the crust to the meat. It also gives your poultry a small protein boost. Crack one open in a shallow bowl, whisk it, and dip the chicken in it. *Tip:* Put your crust ingredients in a shallow plate instead of a bowl—it'll be much easier to coat the breast evenly.

Read 'em and Eat

The fine print on poultry labels

Basted

What it means for the chicken: Up to 8 percent of the meat's weight may come from flavor-enhancing injections or marinades.

What it means for you: Since chicken is sold by weight, you're paying more for less. And those sauces are usually salty. Avoid them.

Free-Range

What it means for the chicken: Foghorn Leghorn can fly the coop anytime he likes.

What it means for you: Since the chicken uses its muscles more often, it will be slightly leaner than a traditionally raised chicken, which spends much of its life packed in a crate with other birds.

Halal

What it means for the chicken: The Quran lays down specific rules for this chicken's slaughter. While humanely cutting the chicken's throat, the Muslim butcher must say the name of Allah.

What it means for you: A lot, if you're a devout Muslim. Otherwise, nothing at all.

Kosher

What it means for the chicken: Jewish religious laws govern the chicken's entire life. Kosher chickens are fed natural grains and slaughtered humanely, and their carcasses are completely drained of blood. (Salt is usually added to help draw it out.)

What it means for you: You're buying a wholesome chicken that's been effectively brined. That means it'll be more moist and tender than ordinary chicken when cooked. It also means that, unless rinsed, the bird can contain a lot of sodium.

Natural

What it means for the chicken: Not much. This term concerns only what happens to the chicken after it's met the Grim Meat Separator—namely, that no artificial colorings have been added.

What it means for you: Zilch.

No Antibiotics

What it means for the chicken: The chicken was raised without the use of antibiotics, which are usually fed to chickens, whether they're sick or not, as a preventive measure.

What it means for you: Dinner won't double as unnecessary medication.

Organic

What it means for the chicken: The chicken was raised according to the USDA's organic rules—no antibiotics, all organic feed, and access to the outdoors.

What it means for you: Chicken as nature intended. Like free-range birds (which are often organic), it's a little leaner than traditional.

25. **Nut crusted:** Dip the chicken in the egg, then roll it in $\frac{1}{3}$ c nuts of your choice, finely chopped. Spray lightly with cooking spray.

26. **Parmesan crusted:** Dip the chicken in the egg, then roll it in a mixture of 1 Tbsp finely grated Parmesan cheese, 1 Tbsp Italian bread crumbs, and a pinch of black pepper.

27. **"Like fried":** Dip the chicken in the egg, then roll it in $\frac{1}{2}$ c crushed cornflakes or bran flakes. Spray lightly with cooking spray.

STUFFED

Relax; this isn't hard. First, pound the heck out of the chicken breast with a meat tenderizer or the heel of your hand— you want it to be uniformly thin. (Just be careful not to tear it.) Then arrange your ingredients on the breast, roll it up, and secure it with toothpicks or kitchen twine so it doesn't come undone while baking.

28. 1 slice Cheddar cheese, 2 slices deli ham, $\frac{1}{4}$ tsp black pepper

29. 1 slice mozzarella cheese; 3 slices pepperoni; 3 leaves fresh basil, chopped

30. 1 slice mozzarella; $\frac{1}{4}$ c chopped tomatoes; 3 leaves fresh basil, chopped

31. 1 small handful baby spinach leaves, chopped; 1 Tbsp blue-cheese crumbles; 1 clove garlic, crushed

32. 1 slice mozzarella, 1 slice salami, 1 Tbsp chopped roasted red pepper

33. $1\frac{1}{2}$ Tbsp part-skim ricotta cheese, 1 Tbsp chopped sun-dried tomatoes, $\frac{1}{4}$ tsp oregano

34. $1\frac{1}{2}$ Tbsp part-skim ricotta cheese, 1 Tbsp diced olives, $\frac{1}{4}$ tsp lemon zest

35. 1 Tbsp pesto, 1 Tbsp grated Parmesan cheese, $\frac{1}{4}$ tsp black pepper

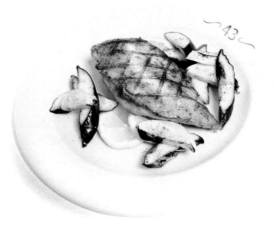

Grilling, Searing, or George Foreman-ing

Basic technique: Heat the grill, place a nonstick skillet over medium-high heat on the stove until it's hot, or power up the Foreman. Add marinated chicken, cooking 3 to 5 minutes per side (6 to 8 total on the Foreman), or until an internal roasting thermometer reaches 170°F. The chicken doesn't stop cooking when you take it off the heat. If it's still hot, it's still cooking.

MARINADES

Marinades need only about an hour or so to penetrate the meat. Whether you're cooking one chicken breast at a time or four at once, just mix the marinade ingredients well in a resealable plastic bag, drop in the chicken, seal, shake, and refrigerate.

Tip: If you're grilling, make a little extra marinade and reserve it in a separate bag or bowl. Brush it on the chicken during cooking to keep the meat moist.

36. 2 Tbsp bourbon, 1 tsp deli-style mustard, ¼ tsp black pepper

37. 2 Tbsp bourbon; 1 tsp honey; 1 clove garlic, crushed

38. 2 Tbsp white wine; 1 clove garlic, crushed; ¼ tsp thyme

39. 2 Tbsp red wine; 1 tsp barbecue sauce; 1 clove garlic, crushed

40. 2 Tbsp Coca-Cola, ¼ tsp black pepper

41. 2 Tbsp balsamic vinaigrette, ¼ tsp rosemary

42. 2 Tbsp lemon juice, ¼ tsp lemon zest, ¼ tsp black pepper

43. 2 Tbsp plain yogurt, ¼ tsp dill

PEAK performance

Fat That Can Make You Lean

New research from Canada shows that taking conjugated linoleic acid (CLA), an omega-6 fatty acid, can make a workout more effective. In a study of 37 men on a 3-day-a-week training program, those who consumed 5 grams (g) of CLA a day built 3 pounds of lean muscle mass, compared with 0.5 pounds for those not taking the supplement. The CLA group also burned more fat. CLA turns on "genes that are responsible for elevating metabolic rate and muscle-cell replication," says lead study author Philip Chilibeck, PhD. Split your dose. The people in the study consumed 2 g with breakfast, 2 g with lunch, and 1 g with supper.

44. 2 Tbsp plain yogurt, 1 tsp olive oil, ¼ tsp curry powder

45. 2 Tbsp lime juice, 1 tsp olive oil, ¼ tsp cilantro

46. 2 Tbsp lime juice, ¼ tsp cumin, ¼ tsp red pepper flakes

47. 2 Tbsp orange juice, ¼ tsp powdered ginger, ¼ tsp cilantro

48. 2 Tbsp orange juice, 1 Tbsp hoisin sauce, ¼ tsp red pepper flakes

49. 1 Tbsp reduced-sodium soy sauce, 1 tsp sesame oil, ¼ tsp red pepper flakes

50. 2 Tbsp pineapple juice; 1 clove garlic, crushed; ¼ tsp black pepper

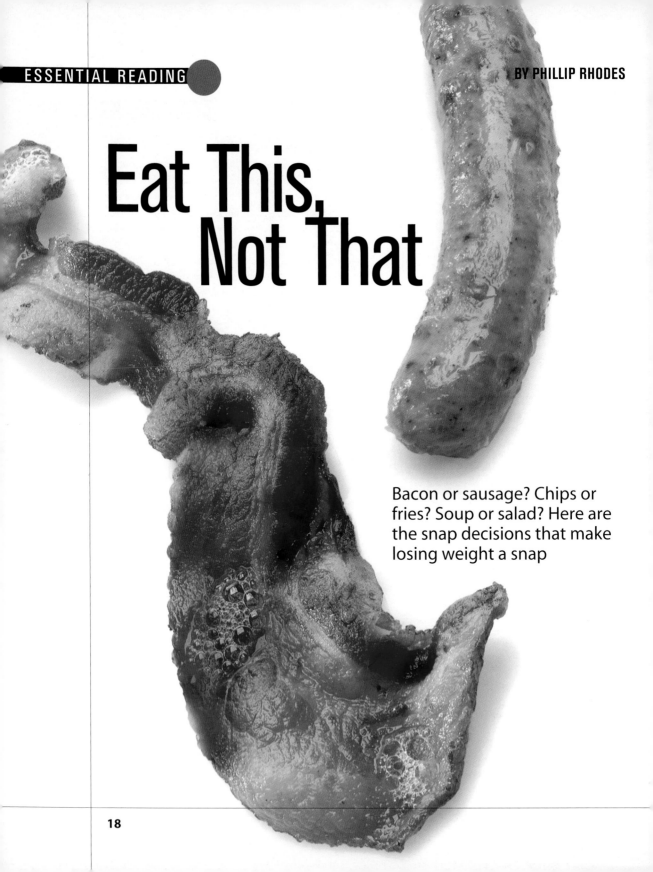

BY PHILLIP RHODES

Eat This, Not That

Bacon or sausage? Chips or fries? Soup or salad? Here are the snap decisions that make losing weight a snap

She smacks her gum, clears her throat, and sighs. We've encountered this impatience in a female plenty of times (11th grade, for starters), but it's especially stressful coming from a waitress. Why can't we answer her simple question: Soup or salad?

If nutrition information would stop advancing, it'd be easy. A couple of years ago, you'd have picked the salad (fat-free ranch on the side, please). Now we know that some vegetables are more nutritious cooked in soup than served raw in salad. And others won't do you much good unless you deliberately pour a fatty dressing on top of them.

So . . . soup it is. Unless it's cream-based; too fatty. And this is just the start of the meal. "Chips or fries?" and "Swiss or Cheddar?" haven't even come up yet. Oh, and "Would you like to see the wine list?"

Time to simplify. We sat down and listed all the pesky mealtime puzzlers we could think of. And then we solved them. No quacks, no product-pushing flacks. Just sensible, easy-to-follow advice that's not likely to change for quite a while—if ever.

At Breakfast

EAT THIS . . .	NOT THAT . . .
Bacon	Sausage
Per slice: 42 calories, 3 grams (g) protein, 0 g carbohydrates, 3 g fat (1 g saturated), 0 g fiber, 192 milligrams (mg) sodium	Per link: 82 calories, 4 g protein, 0 g carbohydrates, 7 g fat (2.6 g saturated), 0 g fiber, 201 mg sodium

The food police were dead wrong when they busted bacon. A crisp slice has about the same amount of protein as a typical pork-sausage link, but half the fat and calories. "For every single sausage link, you could have two pieces of bacon," says Dawn Jackson Blatner, RD, a spokeswoman for the American Dietetic Association. Oh, all right—twist our arm.

EAT THIS . . .	NOT THAT . . .
English muffin	Bagel
Per muffin: 133 calories, 4 g protein, 26 g carbohydrates, 1 g fat (0 g saturated), 1.5 g fiber, 262 mg sodium	Per bagel: 245 calories, 9 g protein, 48 g carbohydrates, 1 g fat (0 g saturated), 2 g fiber, 476 mg sodium

If you're faced with only refined-flour options (as you usually are unless you're breakfasting in Berkeley, California), you can't narrow down these two breads by fiber. So fall back on calories, Blatner advises. "Half a bagel has nearly as many calories as a whole English muffin," she says. "I know it doesn't look any bigger, but it's more dense. All those air pockets in the English muffin are saving you some calories." Enough to justify some jelly.

EAT THIS . . .	NOT THAT . . .
French toast	Belgian waffle
Per 2 slices: 298 calories, 10 g protein, 33 g carbohydrates, 14 g fat (3.5 g saturated), 0 g fiber, 623 mg sodium	Per waffle: 390 calories, 8 g protein, 48 g carbohydrates, 19 g fat (12 g saturated), 1 g fiber, 850 mg sodium

Even though the French toast is dipped in egg batter and lightly fried, the Belgian waffle still outweighs it. "A true Belgian waffle contains a lot of butter and eggs," says Linda Mc-Donald, RD, editor of Supermarket-savvy.com, a food-shopping Web site. "The size is different, too—the waffle is heavier than the French toast." Eat it too often and you'll be heavier, too.

EAT THIS . . .	NOT THAT . . .
Poached egg	**Scrambled egg**
Per egg: 74 calories, 6 g protein, 0 g carbohydrates, 5 g fat (1.5 g saturated), 0 g fiber, 147 mg sodium	Per egg: 101 calories, 7 g protein, 1 g carbohydrates, 7 g fat (2 g saturated), 0 g fiber, 171 mg sodium

"Usually, when you order scrambled eggs, the cook uses butter, oil, or cream to make them," says Blatner. That adds fat and calories. "A poached egg is cooked in water," she says. That adds nothing.

At Lunch

EAT THIS . . .	NOT THAT . . .
Turkey-and-ham wrap	**Turkey-and-ham sub**
Per wrap: 390 calories, 32 g protein, 19 g carbohydrates, 23 g fat (8 g saturated), 9 g fiber, 1,890 mg sodium	Per 6-inch sub: 476 calories, 30 g protein, 52 g carbohydrates, 16 g fat (7 g saturated), 3 g fiber, 1,690 mg sodium

"Typically, with a sub sandwich, you're going to get a colossal roll that might be the equivalent of four to eight pieces of bread but has little fiber," says Dave Grotto, RD, director of nutrition education at the Block Center for Integrative Cancer Care in Evanston, Illinois. Most wraps have 3 to 6 g of fiber—and that's before you factor in the vegetables, which will help cover nearly a third of your daily recommended allowance.

EAT THIS . . .	NOT THAT . . .
Baked beans	**Coleslaw**
Per 6-ounce serving: 230 calories, 8 g protein, 46 g carbohydrates, 1 g fat (1 g saturated), 7 g fiber, 720 mg sodium	Per 6-ounce serving: 190 calories, 1 g protein, 22 g carbohydrates, 11 g fat (2 g saturated), 3 g fiber, 300 mg sodium

"Beans reign supreme in many nutrition categories," especially protein, says Grotto. "Plus, there's no comparison for fiber; beans blow away—sorry for the bad word choice—the coleslaw."

EAT THIS . . .	NOT THAT . . .
Beef burrito	**Beef quesadilla**
Per serving: 440 calories, 17 g protein, 52 g carbohydrates, 18 g fat (8 g saturated), 5 g fiber, 1,330 mg sodium	Per serving: 470 calories, 26 g protein, 38 g carbohydrates, 24 g fat (13 g saturated), 3 g fiber, 1,270 mg sodium

Much like its culinary cousin the wrap sandwich, the burrito leaves more room for good stuff—vegetables that add fiber but not fat. The quesadilla is just meat and cheese—and lots of both.

EAT THIS . . .	NOT THAT . . .
Chips	**Fries**
Per 1-ounce bag: 152 calories, 2 g protein, 15 g carbohydrates, 10 g fat (3 g saturated), 1 g fiber, 168 mg sodium	Per 3-ounce serving: 270 calories, 3 g protein, 34 g carbohydrates, 13 g fat (3 g saturated), 4 g fiber, 115 mg sodium

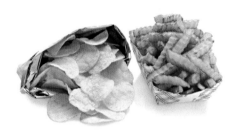

First, there's the serving-size issue. The bag of chips that usually comes with a sandwich has a net weight of 1 ounce. The fries that come with your burger start at 3 ounces. Then there's the fat. Fries, especially crinkle-cut ones, have more surface area, so they soak up more saturated fat from cooking oil. Plus, many processed fries are sprayed with partially hydrogenated fat before they leave the factory. "So it doesn't make a difference what they're fried in; they already contain trans fat," Grotto says.

EAT THIS . . .	NOT THAT . . .
Ground-beef pizza topping	**Pepperoni pizza topping**
Per ounce: 54 calories, 8 g protein, 0 g carbohydrates, 2 g fat (1 g saturated), 0 g fiber, 24 mg sodium	Per ounce: 130 calories, 6 g protein, 1 g carbohydrates, 11 g fat (4.5 g saturated), 0 g fiber, 501 mg sodium

The highest-quality beef doesn't end life as a pizza topping. But ground beef is still a leaner leftover than pepperoni, which is a combination of meat scraps made palatable by the addition of fat and sodium, says McDonald.

At Snack Time

EAT THIS . . .	NOT THAT . . .
Popcorn	**Nachos**
Per 10-cup serving: 550 calories, 10 g protein, 63 g carbohydrates, 31 g fat (5 g saturated), 11 g fiber, 972 mg sodium	Per serving (6 to 8 nachos): 608 calories, 17 g protein, 60 g carbohydrates, 34 g fat (14 g saturated), 2 g fiber, 1,736 mg sodium

Ballpark or movie-theater popcorn—even when it's popped in oil and sprayed with "butter"—outranks the Mexican fare. "The popcorn is not a low-cal food by any means," says Blatner, "but it does give you 11 g of fiber." But nachos have cheese, which is good, right? Uh, not if it's poured on from a dispenser. "That stuff isn't cheese," she says. It's just trans fatty orange goo.

EAT THIS . . .	NOT THAT . . .
Salsa	**Guacamole**
Per 2 tablespoons: 9 calories, 1 g protein, 2 g carbohydrates, 0 g fat, 1 g fiber, 198 mg sodium	Per 2 tablespoons: 55 calories, 0 g protein, 2 g carbohydrates, 5 g fat (0 g saturated), 0 g fiber, 126 mg sodium

"Guys ask me this one all the time," says Blatner. "They'll say, 'I just read that guacamole has good fat.' It does. But, for your prostate, you should probably have the salsa. It has lycopene [1,700 micrograms, or 10 percent of the amount you need daily]."

EAT THIS . . .	NOT THAT . . .
Swiss	Cheddar
Per ounce: 108 calories, 8 g protein, 2 g carbohydrates, 8 g fat (5 g saturated), 0 g fiber, 54 mg sodium	Per ounce: 114 calories, 7 g protein, 0 g carbohydrates, 9 g fat (6 g saturated), 0 g fiber, 176 mg sodium

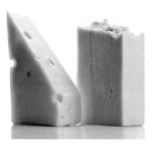

When it comes to sodium, ounce for ounce, Cheddar has three times more of the salty stuff than Swiss. No, one slice won't cause you to have a stroke on the spot. But when you're faced with the burger-topping choice, it's good to know.

At Dinner

EAT THIS . . .	NOT THAT . . .
Minestrone	Salad (with 2 tablespoons blue cheese dressing)
Per 1½-cup serving: 184 calories, 7 g protein, 31 g carbohydrates, 4 g fat (1 g saturated), 2 g fiber, 705 mg sodium	Per 1½-cup serving: 184 calories, 4 g protein, 9 g carbohydrates, 16 g fat (3 g saturated), 1 g fiber, 328 mg sodium

"Most side salads are just iceberg lettuce, which is mostly water and no nutrients," says McDonald. "If the soup has lots of vegetables and a clear broth, it would be the better choice." The vegetables are cooked, re-

leasing nutrients and making them easier for your body to absorb. (Cheddar-broccoli soup doesn't count.)

EAT THIS . . .	NOT THAT . . .
Balsamic vinaigrette	Blue cheese dressing
Per 2 tablespoons: 60 calories, 0 g protein, 3 g carbohydrates, 5 g fat (0.5 g saturated), 0 g fiber, 280 mg sodium	Per 2 tablespoons: 160 calories, 0 g protein, 2 g carbohydrates, 17 g fat (2.5 g saturated), 0 g fiber, 260 mg sodium

Still want a salad instead of soup? That's okay. Dress yours with vinaigrette. Why? All the flavor (courtesy of the tangy vinegar), for a fraction of the fat and calories. You'll also avoid a gram or two of trans fats, which most creamy packaged dressings contain.

EAT THIS . . .	NOT THAT . . .
Baked potato	Rice pilaf
Per medium potato: 161 calories, 4 g protein, 37 g carbohydrates, 0 g fat, 4 g fiber, 17 mg sodium	Per 1-cup serving: 220 calories, 5 g protein, 44 g carbohydrates, 4 g fat (2 g saturated), 1 g fiber, 820 mg sodium

You can't keep a good carb down. Since the rice could have anything in it—a tub of butter or salty stock—opt for the much-maligned tuber. "Just make sure you eat the skin—that's where the fiber is," Blatner says.

EAT THIS . . .	NOT THAT . . .
Grilled salmon	Grilled skinless chicken breast
Per 3-ounce serving: 175 calories, 19 g protein, 0 g carbohydrates, 11 g fat (2 g saturated), 0 g fiber, 52 mg sodium	Per 3-ounce serving: 142 calories, 27 g protein, 0 g carbohydrates, 3 g fat (1 g saturated), 0 g fiber, 64 mg sodium

The chicken isn't a bad choice—it has fewer calories, less fat, more protein, and doesn't have salmon's slightly cloudy environmental reputation. But the chicken doesn't have salmon's healthful omega-3 fats. "What salmon brings to the table in the way of omega-3 fats far outweighs the concern about added fat and calories," says Grotto. Omega-3s fight the number one killer of men: heart disease. "Even the debate about whether to choose wild or farm-raised, or avoid salmon altogether because of PCB concerns, is still overshadowed by the positive health attributes of this fish," he says.

EAT THIS . . .	NOT THAT . . .
Hot fudge sundae	**Cheesecake**
Per 1/2-cup serving: 284 calories, 6 g protein, 48 g carbohydrates, 9 g fat (5 g saturated), 0 g fiber, 182 mg sodium, 207 mg calcium	Per piece: 257 calories, 4 g protein, 20 g carbohydrates, 18 g fat (8 g saturated), 0 g fiber, 166 mg sodium, 41 mg calcium

Two dairy desserts. But only one gives you nuts, chocolate sauce, and an impressive amount of fat-burning calcium.

DRINK THIS . . .	NOT THAT . . .
Tomato juice	**Orange juice**
Per 8 ounces low-sodium juice: 53 calories, 1 g protein, 11 g carbohydrates, 0 g fat, 2 g fiber, 169 mg sodium	Per 8 ounces: 109 calories, 2 g protein, 25 g carbohydrates, 1 g fat, 1 g fiber, 2 mg sodium

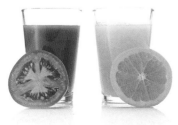

This isn't a matter of the lesser of two evils; it's the greater of two goods. "Both are high in vitamin C, which may fight cardiovascular disease. But the tomato juice is high in lycopene," says Grotto. "I would lean toward tomato juice." The two nutrients address the biggest health concerns for men—prostate cancer and heart disease.

DRINK THIS . . .	NOT THAT . . .
Red wine	**White wine**
Per 3.5-ounce glass: 74 calories, 0 g protein, 2 g carbohydrates, 0 g fat, 0 g fiber, 5 mg sodium	Per 3.5-ounce glass: 70 calories, 0 g protein, 1 g carbohydrates, 0 g fat, 0 g fiber, 5 mg sodium

"Red wine is better than white on the antioxidant front," says Karen MacNeil, author of the encyclopedic reference *The Wine Bible*. According to a recent study at the University of Barcelona in Spain, red wine can reduce the markers of inflammation by 21 percent. Credit grape skins, which contain the antioxidants that give red wine both its color and its health benefits.

TOUGH TALK

"Avoid any diet that discourages the use of hot fudge."
DON KARDONG, 1976 U.S. OLYMPIC MARATHONER

BY TIMOTHY GOWER

Shake Off the Weight

No calorie counting, no carb watching. For half a century, meal-replacement shakes have been a no-brainer way to drop pounds. Why? They work

For Rob Nager, the epiphany occurred at Abercrombie & Fitch. He was picking through a stack of cargo pants and asked a clerk if they were available in a 42-inch waist. "Dude," the kid sneered, "we don't *make* pants that big."

Nager, 38, faced a choice. He could ask the little weasel to step outside, or he could do

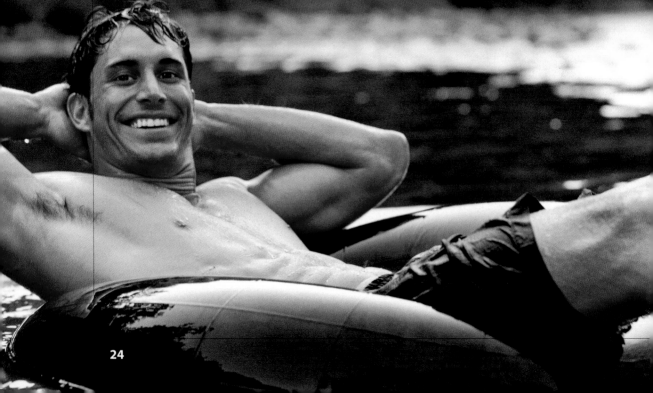

something about his 250-pound frame. He opted for peace and a new waistline.

He tried Weight Watchers, then Atkins. Both plans helped him slim down, but the flab always returned. Finally, Nager tried a weight-loss strategy that's been around since TVs were black-and-white; a strategy so old-school that one of the studies showing that it works went on for a decade. His throwback approach: meal-replacement beverages (MRs, in the weight-loss world). Nager just said no to solid food. Instead, he quaffed shakes in place of meals, eventually losing 22 pounds. That was 2 years ago. The weight is still off.

The Proof Is in the Paunch

They're simple and they're foolproof. That's why MRs work for men who are too busy to worry about calories, says Allan Geliebter, PhD, a research psychologist at the New York Obesity Research Center at St. Luke's–Roosevelt Hospital in Manhattan. "They just know that this is what they consume, and they don't have to think too much about it," says Geliebter. The best candidate for liquid lunches (and breakfasts), he says, is a guy who's healthy but wants to drop 10 to 20 pounds.

MRs come in two basic forms: liquid-only programs administered by physicians and the more familiar over-the-counter products sold in groceries and drugstores. The prescribed plans (like Optifast and HMR) replace all meals and are usually for seriously overweight patients. We'll focus on the over-the-counter options, like Slim-Fast, Met-Rx, and GNC. They contain about 200 calories per serving, plus a dose of vitamins and minerals, and they're typically used to replace one or two meals a day. Most are available in ready-to-drink cans or powder packets that can be mixed with water or milk.

A few years ago, Steven Heymsfield, MD, also of St. Luke's–Roosevelt, analyzed a half-dozen small studies comparing Slim-Fast with conventional low-calorie diets. He found that people who guzzle the shakes in place of one or two meals a day consistently lose 7 to 8 percent of their body weight after 1 year. That's about 15 pounds for a 200-pound man, which, he notes, is roughly the same reduction you might achieve by taking a weight-loss drug such as Xenical—minus the risk of a drug's side effects (which include such horrors as "oily stools"). Meanwhile, Dr. Heymsfield showed that people who simply try to eat less maintain a weight loss closer to 3 percent.

Pretty impressive, but most of the studies Dr. Heymsfield analyzed lasted only a year. Any obesity doctor worth his fat calipers knows that anyone can lose a few pounds, but keeping that weight off over the long term is far more difficult.

So how about a 10-year study? That's right. George Blackburn, MD, an expert in nutrition and metabolism at Harvard

HARD TRUTH

Run It Off

Number of miles you'd have to run to burn the 1,200 calories in 1 pint of Ben & Jerry's Chunky Monkey ice cream:

13.4

(the length of Manhattan Island)

Medical School, released findings from a study comparing two groups of people in the aptly named town of Pound, Wisconsin. The Harvard team gave one group Slim-Fast, with instructions to replace two meals a day with the shakes in an effort to shed pounds. When they reached their goal weights, the Slim-Fast folks were encouraged to keep pounds off by replacing one meal per day with a shake. The comparison group simply "followed the eating habits of their community," says Dr. Blackburn—which, in Wis-

We Drank It, We Ranked It

If these shakes are replacing meals, they'd better taste good

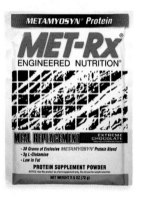

1. MET-Rx
Thick and chocolatey—like a real milkshake. A very filling 16 ounces.

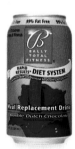

2. Bally
More malt than chocolate, but that's not a bad thing.

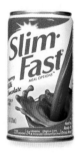

3. Slim-Fast
Great flavor at first, but a slightly bitter vitamin aftertaste. A bit grainy.

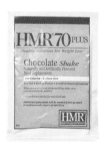

4. HMR 70 Plus
A 6-ounce shake isn't much of a meal. Complicated mixing process, too.

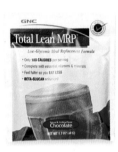

5. GNC Total Lean MRP
Strange alcohol taste—like a bad Kahlúa drink. Slightly grainy.

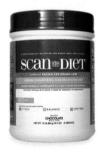

6. Scan Diet
Watery texture with a taste more wheat field than chocolate. Stay away.

consin, likely included lots of cheese and bratwurst.

A decade later, the men using Slim-Fast had maintained a 7-pound weight loss, on average. Big deal, right? Well, yes, when you consider that their cheesehead counterparts gained 25 pounds, on average, during that same 10-year stretch.

Shake It Off

So why do meal-replacement diets work? Mathematics, mostly. "There's nothing magical about the shakes. Weight loss is a function of calories in, calories out," says clinical psychologist Anthony Fabricatore, PhD, of the University of Pennsylvania weight and eating-disorders program.

To wit: An 11-ounce can of Slim-Fast Creamy Milk Chocolate contains 220 calories. Swap one for your daily lunch—say, a beef burrito and large cola, which weighs in at 600 calories—and eventually you'll start subtracting numbers on your bathroom scale.

Companies that peddle MRs on the Internet often claim exotic "fat-burning!" ingredients. Experts scoff, but there is evidence that the main ingredient in most MRs—nonfat milk—may battle the bulge. According to University of Tennessee nutritionist Michael Zemel, PhD, author of *The Calcium Key*, calcium suppresses a hormone that signals the body to make bigger fat cells and burn less blubber, while amino acids in dairy foods further promote the breakdown

of fat cells while preserving muscle. "On a dairy-rich diet, you lose more fat and less lean tissue," he says.

At first, many MR users feel hungry. But this will fade fast—most MRs have plenty of protein and fiber to forestall a pantry raid. Forgoing the pleasures of mastication, however, can be harder. Nager, who initially enrolled in a medically supervised liquid-only diet plan, says, "After a while, I was losing my mind. I needed to chew." So he did, reintroducing solid food into his diet once he'd gotten his weight under control.

How long does this kind of diet last? As long as you want it to. Some patients stay on only until the weight comes off. Others, like Nager, stay on, to some degree, for life. "Data imply that one meal replacement per day can be used long-term," says Fabricatore, who recommends regular consultation with a licensed nutritionist if you plan on using two MRs per day for more than 5 months.

Nager says he doesn't miss the three-square-meals-a-day life; in fact, he says he's happy not to be constantly worried about food anymore. "If I stop my routine, I'm going to get hungry," he says. "Then I'd start slipping back into my old habits. This is a deal I'm willing to make." His weight loss has had a domino effect. Not only has he become a fitness fanatic, but Nager quit his high-pressure job in corporate sales and started a dog-walking business. "I feel better; I look better," he says.

Training Tips

I work from midnight to 8:00 A.M. When should I eat and work out?

E.G., MAUMEE, OHIO

Do what 9-to-5ers do, but back it up 9 hours. Eat breakfast at 11:00 P.M. to start up your metabolism. Have a snack around 1:00 A.M. and lunch at 4:00 A.M. You should work out after you're off the clock, so eat some fruit or yogurt around 6:00 A.M. to make sure you have energy for exercise. Finally, have dinner around 11:00 A.M. and a bedtime snack around 1:00 P.M. so you'll sleep well when you hit the sack at around 2:00.

PET PROJECT

Run with Spot

There's scientific proof that people look like their dogs: A recent study found that when both people and pets went on a diet and took walks together, both lost weight. Take General Patton on a stroll farther than the backyard to do his business. If you're canine deficient, adopt a best friend. Or offer to walk your cute neighbor's pooch. You dog, you.

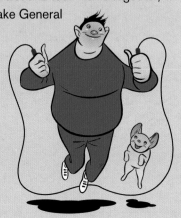

WEIGH YOUR OPTIONS

When I'm stuck at work, what's better: eating junk from the vending machine or not eating at all?

T.L., DENVER

I believe you should eat when you're truly hungry. Look for the healthiest option available—trail mix or the candy bar with the most nuts in it to fill you up. Going hungry could just make you eat more later and do more damage. The best strategy: Stash snacks (granola bars, almonds, peanut butter, dried soup mix) in your desk so you have healthy options handy.

LIQUID GOLD

What's the best liquid to use in a protein shake?

T.A., FLANDERS, NEW JERSEY

Milk. "Dairy products aid in fat loss," says Mary Ellen Camire, PhD, a professor of food science and human nutrition at the University of Maine and a member of the *Men's Health* Advisory Board. If you're lactose intolerant, try Lactaid or Dairy Ease brands, which can be found in most grocery stores. Use shakes as a vessel to carry aboard the much-needed food group—you'll get the muscle-building power of protein along with fat-fighting calcium, while improving bone and cardiovascular health to boot.

SWEET THING

Should I be concerned about the high-fructose corn syrup I see in the ingredients of some meal-replacement bars?

S.L., PEACHTREE CITY, GEORGIA

Not necessarily. If you're exercising strenuously or if you're trying to bulk up, high-fructose corn syrup isn't terrible. But if you want to cut calories or carbs, you should avoid this processed sugar. Look for natural sweeteners like fruit juice, molasses, or evaporated cane juice.

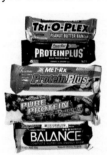

FREE FROM WORRY?

Have there been any proven long-term side effects from taking ephedra-free Hydroxycut?

R.H., PROVIDENCE, RHODE ISLAND

It's tough to say for sure. Hydroxycut has at least 11 active ingredients, and ephedra may not have been the only problematic one. Chromium, just one of the other active ingredients, is a good example. Doses of more than 600 micrograms a day of chromium have been associated with liver and kidney failure, among other serious health risks. So there's no bottom line on how safe Hydroxycut is—even without ephedra. Your best bet is to consult your physician before trying it.

TIME WELL SPENT

I have an hour every morning. Should I do cardio or weight lifting to boost my metabolism?

T.M., LANDOVER, MARYLAND

Alternate between the two. You'll likely burn more calories in an hour of aerobics than you would during an hour of weight lifting. But weight lifting makes you burn more calories between workouts.

CUT YOUR LOSSES

How do I know if I'm losing fat or muscle?

K.J., ST. PAUL, MINNESOTA

You're probably losing both. Some muscle loss occurs along with any weight loss, but strength training helps limit the amount. Use a scale that measures body fat to monitor your body composition. But it will take 6 to 8 weeks to see a change.

Less Booze, You Lose

If you're looking to lose weight, order the gin and tonic without the gin. Alcohol lowers your body's ability to burn fat by as much as 36 percent.

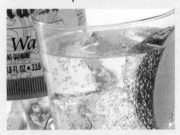

HARD HABIT TO BREAK

I kicked my pretzel habit, but now I suck on hard candy. Which is worse?

M.K., LITTLE ROCK, ARKANSAS

You're probably taking in fewer calories by snacking on candy rather than pretzels. But it sounds as if you're eating for reasons other than hunger. Keep a stress ball and a glass of water at your desk instead of snacks.

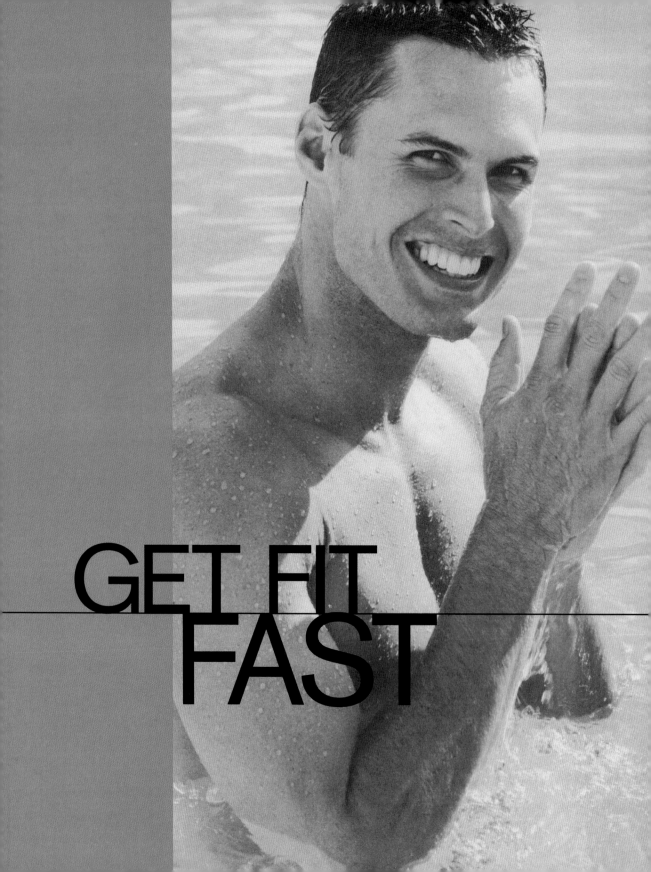

GET FIT
FAST

Kenneth Cooper, MD, founder and director of the renowned Cooper Aerobics Center in Dallas, has been quoted as saying, "The average American takes 20 years to get out of condition and he wants to get back in condition in 20 days—and you just can't do it."

The good doctor's right, of course. But at *Men's Health*, we've never settled for being just average. Which is why we put together the fastest get-fit plan you'll find anywhere. Sure, it may take more than 20 days to get fit—even with our plan—and especially if your only form of exercise has been getting up from the couch to get a beer. Still, we'd like you to take the challenge—follow any one of the workouts in this section for the next 20 days and see what happens. We guarantee you'll be well on your way to getting into the best shape of your life.

Start by taking our test to find out where you are now and where you need to go. Then learn how to design your workout around *your* fitness goals, streamline time wasters from your routine, and get total-body results—fast. We even tackle the top excuses that derail the best-intentioned guys from their fitness programs.

Now that you have no excuses, what are you waiting for? Your 20 days to a better body start today.

BY LARA ROSENBAUM

The Five Pillars of Fitness

A balanced workout achieves strength, power, endurance, agility, and flexibility. Here's the only plan you'll need this year

How fit are you?

Right now, you probably do two types of training: strength and cardiovascular. Great if you want to look ripped and run long, but lousy if you want to be able to legitimately call yourself fit.

Consider a top athlete like Terrell Owens. By incorporating plyometrics and agility work into his training, he's able to twist, jump, and juke his way past angry NFL officials. And because he stretches, too, he's less likely to injure himself while sprinting across the goal line. Or doing pushups in the end zone. Not to mention he's better able to return to the game in record time if he ever does get injured.

Of course, you're no T.O. But if

you build your workout around these same five pillars—strength, cardio, flexibility, agility, and power—you can reach your peak fitness years, just as he has.

First step: Pull out a Sharpie or other fine writing implement and take our fitness test. It'll help you design a five-tool workout that can get you in your best shape ever this year—and this lifetime. And that's cause for celebration (with no penalty).

Directions: These tests will assess your baseline fitness in the five core areas. When you're finished, write down your results. That'll guide you in putting together your custom workout from the pages that follow. Retest yourself every 4 to 6 weeks to see where you're moving and where you're mired. Then make instant adjustments to kick-start your fitness.

PILLAR 1: STRENGTH

Pushups: Drop and give us as many as possible until failure. Maintain proper form throughout. If you cheat, you're done.

Scoring: Top army recruits do 68 pushups in 2 minutes. Your upper body is buff if you can grunt out 40 to 50 in that time.

Situps: Lie with your feet flat on the floor, your knees bent 90 degrees, and your hands resting on your thighs. Curl your torso up, sliding your hands toward your knees, then lower yourself back down. Perform as many as you can in 1 minute, while keeping your feet on the floor.

Scoring: A score of 40 repetitions per minute (rpm) is a sign of a solid core. The average for most men is 35 rpm.

Squats: Keeping your knees behind your toes and your torso straight, bend your knees and lower yourself until your thighs are parallel to the floor. Slowly stand back up and repeat. Continue until failure or until you break form.

Scoring: Do the old up-and-down 31 to 34 times and your leg strength is average. Close in on 45 times and it's excellent.

PILLAR 2: CARDIOVASCULAR FITNESS

3-Minute Step Test: Find a 12- to 18-inch step or sturdy box. Keep a consistent four-beat pace while you step up and down for 3 minutes straight. Rest for 1 minute, then take your pulse for 30 seconds. Multiply the result by 5.6 and divide this into 18,000 (the duration of exercise in seconds multiplied by 100). This is your step-test score.

Scoring: The higher your step-test score, the more efficient your body's blood pump. Anything between 60 and 100 is considered fit.

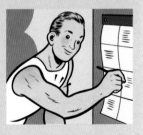

PEAK
performance

Put It in Writing

Instead of waiting to see results in the mirror, look for the payoff on paper. Every time you exercise or lift weights, write down what you've done, suggests motivational expert Robert Burns. "Seeing your day-to-day progress on paper is a powerful inspiration to continue your work," he explains. A good way to keep track of your efforts: Write your daily accomplishments on a calendar. Realizing you can do 10 more reps today than you could last week will keep you going back for more.

PILLAR 3: FLEXIBILITY

Sit and Reach: Put a 12-inch ruler on top of a box so that half of it is hanging off. Now sit on the floor with your legs extended and your bare feet flat against the front of the box and on either side of the ruler. With hands overlapping and legs straight, lean forward as far as you can. Hold your stretch and note the distance between your fingertips and toes. (Negative numbers if you stop before your feet, positive if you reach beyond.)

Scoring: If you can stretch 2 to 6 inches past your feet, you're flexible. More than 6 inches and you're downright elastic.

PEAK
performance

Drink Up

Once the weather warms up, remember: Your muscles need H_2O to work at peak efficiency. By the time your brain tells you you're thirsty, your body's fluids are depleted, says Larry Kenney, PhD, president of the American College of Sports Medicine, so start drinking water at least 15 minutes before beginning your activity. The rule of thumb is to drink 8 ounces of water for every 20 minutes of exercise.

You can also weigh yourself before and after a workout, and subtract the weight of any water you drank while exercising. For every pound of body weight you lost during the workout, drink 16 ounces of water. Then remember that guideline for your next workout. So if you're 2 pounds lighter after an hour-long run, drink

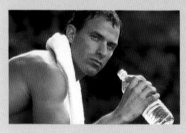

32 ounces more before or during your next run. Sound like more than you can swallow? Kenney says some people find that they can drink more of a sports drink than of water.

PILLAR 4: AGILITY

Shuttle Run: Place two strips of tape 3 yards apart and set two light books beyond the far strip, which we'll call mark #2. Standing on mark #1, time the following sequence.

1. (Start watch.) Sprint to mark #2; grab a book.

2. Sprint back to #1 and place the book right behind the tape.

3. Sprint back to #2 to grab the second book and return to #1, stopping your watch as you pass it.

Scoring: Under 10 seconds is speedy. Under 9 is practically supersonic—the fastest men run the shuttle in 8.7 seconds.

PILLAR 5: POWER (PLYOMETRIC ABILITY)

Vertical Jump: Wet the fingers of your right hand and stand with your right side touching a wall. Reach up with your right hand and mark the highest point you can touch. Now rewet your fingers and stand next to the wall again. This time, jump with both legs and extend your right arm to touch the wall. Jump three times and note your highest mark. Your vertical leap is the difference in inches between your standing reach and your top jump mark.

Scoring: The magic number is 20 inches. Sky that high and your springs are in great shape.

The Five Pillars Workout Plan

Maybe you flunked our fitness tests. Or perhaps you aced all of them (in which case, we know you cheated). But odds are you fell somewhere in the middle of the bell curve of buffness. And really, that's what we expected, which is why we're now going to do something your teachers never did: hand over the answers to next month's tests. The answers, of course, are exercises. Each of the five pillars of fitness has its own selection of exercises, which can be mixed and matched to make a complete week of workouts. Simply follow the training prescriptions that correspond to your test scores, and your new body will follow.

STRENGTH TRAINING

Why you need it: Because weakness is for wimps. Still, strength training isn't just about counting off biceps curls; you also need functional exercises—moves that work the body in its full range of motion and incorporate balance and stability factors. Think of functional training as "movement rehearsal," says Juan Carlos Santana, CSCS, director of the Institute of Human Performance in Boca Raton, Florida. "You need to 'rehearse' natural patterns to build usable strength and protect yourself from injuries."

If you scored . . .

. . . less than 40 in two or more of the strength tests: Train for 30 minutes three times a week. Start with light weights and do three sets of 12 repetitions of each exercise, resting for 1½ minutes between sets.

. . . 40 or higher in two or more of the strength tests: Train for 30 minutes three times a week, but use a weight that's challenging (you can complete your reps, but

Schedule Your New Body
A sample weeklong workout plan for your PDA

Monday
5 minutes flexibility
30 minutes strength
5 minutes flexibility
Total time: 40 minutes

Tuesday
30 minutes cardio
10 minutes agility
Total time: 40 minutes

Wednesday
5 minutes flexibility
10 minutes plyometrics
30 minutes strength
5 minutes flexibility
Total time: 50 minutes

Thursday
5 minutes flexibility
30 minutes cardio (including agility training)
5 minutes flexibility
Total time: 40 minutes

Friday
30 minutes cardio (including 10 minutes plyometrics)
30 minutes strength
Total time: 60 minutes

Saturday
60 minutes cardio
Total time: 60 minutes

Sunday Off

Note: If you have time, add flexibility work to the days where it's missing. Ideally, you'll do it every time you work out.

you have to really push it at the end). If you don't want to give up your current strength routine, incorporate at least three functional moves (any of the "chops") into your workouts.

The Exercises

In addition to functional moves that work several muscle groups at once, we've included a modified crunch, pushup, and dumbbell row for when you want to target specific muscle groups. You can mix and match the exercises however you want, but be sure to work each muscle group at least once during the week.

Diagonal Chop Hold a 6- to 8-pound medicine ball or plate in front of your chest and stand with your feet shoulder-width apart. Pivot on your right foot and rotate 90 degrees to the right, while raising the ball up and to the right. Make sure to keep your left knee aligned with your toes to prevent it from twisting. Next, pivot on your left foot and bring the ball down toward that foot. That's one repetition. Do 10 reps, then switch sides.

Vertical Chop Raise a 6- to 8-pound medicine ball straight above your head and stand with your feet shoulder-width apart. Chop down between your legs with the medicine ball, but don't let it touch the floor. Keep your hips, knees, and feet aligned as you would for a squat. Do 10 to 12 repetitions.

Reaching Lunge Chop to Overhead Reach Stand holding a medicine ball over your

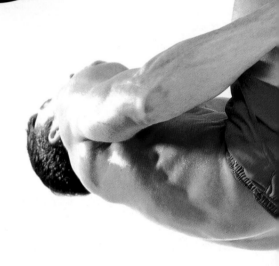

head with your arms straight. Lunge forward and bring the ball to the instep of your front foot. Pause when your back knee is about an inch off the floor, then push back to the starting position. Do a set of 10 reps with one leg before lunging with the other.

Weighted Cross Crunch Lie on your back on the floor and hold a dumbbell or medicine ball with both hands near your right shoulder. Curl your torso up and to the left as you bring the weight to the left of your left hip. Do 10 reps, then repeat the move to the right.

Swiss-Ball Pushup Assume the standard pushup position, but rest your hands directly

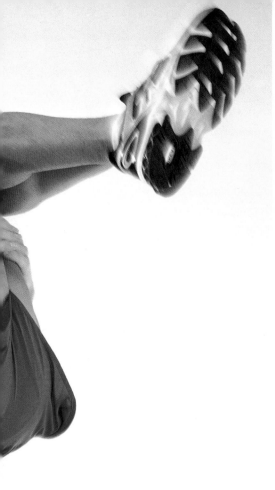

under your shoulders on a Swiss ball and your toes on the floor. Bend your arms until your chest touches the ball. Pause, then push yourself back up to the starting position. Do 10 repetitions.

Staggered-Stance Dumbbell Row Grab a pair of dumbbells and stand with your right foot a couple of feet in front of your left. Bend forward at the hips until your back is at a 45-degree angle to the floor. Keep your back straight. Now pull the weights up to your chest, pause, and slowly lower them back down. Do 10 reps, then do another set with your left foot forward. For a greater challenge, lift your back leg off the floor and

balance on your front leg during the exercise. Lower your torso until it's parallel to the floor. Then do the row.

Plateau Buster Amp up your intensity by adding more weight. And try supplementing every other session with balance work. For example, you might turn two-legged exercises (such as squats) into one-legged versions or train on an unstable surface, like a foam pad or a balance disk.

CARDIOVASCULAR TRAINING

Why you need it: Regular cardio conditions your heart to pump more blood with each contraction, providing your body with extra energy and endurance. Upping your heart rate also burns calories, which directly translates to less fat and more-visible abs. And don't worry about losing muscle mass from excessive calorie burn; your body will need to churn through 2,000 grams of glycogen before it dips into your protein stores, which, if you're running, doesn't happen until about mile 20. *Note:* Before you proceed, estimate your maximum heart rate (MHR) by subtracting your age from 220.

If you scored ...

... lower than 60 in the step test: Do 30 to 60 minutes of low-intensity training four times a week. (Low intensity is defined as 65 percent of your MHR.) You can walk, hike, jog, bike, swim—anything, as long as it's continuous. Gradually increase your intensity to between 70 and 75 percent of your MHR over the next 4 to 6 weeks, and start incorporating some of the interval workouts we provide below.

...60 or higher in the step test: Train at varying levels of intensity for 30 to 60 minutes four times a week. That means going from low intensity (65 percent of your MHR) to moderate intensity (70 percent) to high intensity (at least 85 percent) throughout the week. You can also mix all three levels in one session by doing an interval workout.

The Workouts

These interval workouts are some of the personal favorites of Tom Holland, CSCS, a physiologist and triathlete in Darien, Connecticut. Translation: They're tough. Make sure you warm up with 5 to 10 minutes of easy cardiovascular work, such as jogging in place. Do two or three each week in place of ordinary runs and switch them up to keep your body challenged.

Random Intervals, aka the Traffic Game Start with leisurely running, biking, or inline skating. When a car passes, sprint and see how long you can keep up with the car. Hol-

land chases traffic to break up the monotony of regular runs. Continue for a half hour to an hour, depending on your pace.

Random Intervals, aka the Jam Session Make an MP3 or iPod mix with music of different tempos. When the rhythm is fast, increase your pace to keep up with it. When the music slows down, do the same. (The length of the training session depends on the speed of your songs.)

Hill-Sprint Intervals Sprint up a hill and jog back down. Holland suggests measuring your pulse at the bottom. You'll know you're getting fitter when you can get your heart rate lower and lower. Continue for 15 minutes.

Negative Splits Run or bike at moderate intensity for 15 minutes, then increase your speed and intensity for 15 more. Or, if you're outside, run or bike a half mile, then turn around and sprint back to your starting point. Gradually increase the distance as you improve.

Intervals Jog easily for 10 minutes to warm up, then sprint hard for 2 minutes. Walk for 1 minute, then sprint for 2 more. Repeat the sequence three times, then jog for 10 minutes to recover. For variety, try this interval plan on your bike or in the pool.

Plateau Buster Push your intensity up a notch by sprinting longer or farther. You can also knock off two cardio training sessions in a row and reap more fat loss. "The real fun comes after the first half hour," Holland says. "You begin to destress and experience flow. You'll actually want to exercise longer."

FLEXIBILITY TRAINING

Why you need it:

Stretching increases your range of motion and helps keep you from getting sidelined. "Most injuries result from a decreased range of motion," says Micheal A. Clark, DPT, MS, PT, CEO of the National Academy of Sports Medicine and a consultant for the Phoenix Suns. In fact, when the team added Clark's flexibility and corrective exercises to the Suns' fitness routines, their annual injury rate plummeted by 25 percent. Increased pliability may also mean greater muscle efficiency. So maximize your muscles' flexibility and you'll increase strength and power.

If you scored . . .

. . . less than 2 inches in the sit and reach:

Do 10 minutes of stretching three times a week. Choose from the stretches below, and try to split that time between preworkout dynamic stretches to warm up your muscles and postworkout static stretches to cool them off.

. . . more than 2 inches in the sit and reach:

Same as above, except do static stretches only for the muscles you're training that day.

The Stretches

These stretches focus on your calves, hip flexors, abductors, and lats—muscles, Clark says, that are usually tight. Take it easy on your hamstrings, though. "They're often sore from being overworked," he says, "but that doesn't necessarily mean they're tight."

HARD TRUTH

Flex Your Muscle

Percentage of men who work out to become more flexible:

43

Static Stretches

Hold each stretch for 30 seconds.

Calf Stretch Stand facing a wall with the toes of your right foot pressed against the wall and your left foot's toes about a foot behind. Place your hands against the wall. Keeping your body upright, slowly lean forward until you feel a stretch in your left calf. After doing this with both legs, repeat the stretch with your knees slightly bent to stretch the soleus, a muscle deep within the calf.

Iliotibial-Band (Abductor) Stretch Grab a foam roll (available at MensHealth.com/foam), place it on the floor, and lie on your left side so that your left hip is on the roll. Support yourself on your left elbow. Bend your right knee about 90 degrees and place your right foot on the floor. Drag your body against the foam until the roll is just above your knee, then move back again. Hold for 30 seconds at any particularly tight spots, then switch sides.

Hip-Flexor Stretch Stand with your right foot a couple of feet in front of your left foot. Keeping your right foot still, pivot your left foot so that its toes face to the right. Keeping your torso upright, press your left hip forward until you feel a stretch. Hold for 30 seconds, then return to the starting position and repeat with your other leg.

Kneeling Lat Stretch Kneel in front of a chair and grab the seat with one hand. Round your lower back and move your body backward until you feel a stretch in your latissimus dorsi (in your midback, just below your arms). Hold for 30 seconds, then switch arms and repeat.

Dynamic Stretches

Walking Lunge with Twist Stand with your hands clasped against your chest. Step forward with your right foot into a lunge and twist your head and shoulders to the right. (Your hips should face forward throughout the move.) Reverse the movement to push back to the starting position, then lunge with your left foot and twist to the left. Perform 10 lunges with each leg.

Overhead Squat to Calf Raise Stand with your feet shoulder-width apart and your arms straightened overhead. Lower your body until your thighs are parallel to the floor, then push back up and rise onto the balls of your feet at the top of the move. Do 10 repetitions.

Medicine-Ball Rotation Stand with your feet shoulder-width apart and hold a medicine ball close to your chest. Keeping your right foot stationary, pivot your left foot and rotate your torso 90 degrees to the right. (Keep the ball at your chest.) Then pivot your right foot and rotate your torso 180 degrees to the left. Repeat for a total of 10 rotations in each direction.

Plateau Buster Perform additional moves from the static-stretch menu after each workout. (You can also add more reps of the dynamic ones during your warmup.) If a muscle or joint consistently feels tight, see a doctor to rule out an injury.

AGILITY TRAINING

Why you need it: It makes you faster— and gets your game on. "You're quickly changing directions, and the sudden change in force speeds up your reaction time and builds stability," says Chuck Wolf, CSCS, manager of Sport Science and Human Performance at the USA Triathlon National Training Center in Clermont, Florida. Most agility drills work your body in multiple planes, increasing your calorie burn, too. A study published in *Medicine and Science in Sports and Exercise* found that backward movement burns significantly more calories than forward movement does, and lateral motion burns twice as many as forward. "You're expending more energy because you're using muscles that are undertrained," says study author Henry Williford, PhD.

If you scored . . .

. . . more than 10 seconds in the shuttle run: Complete 5 minutes of agility training twice a week.

. . . 10 seconds or less in the shuttle run: Shoot for 10 minutes of agility training twice a week.

The Drills

Plug agility drills into your warmup to increase your heart rate and work your body in different directions. You can also throw a few into your cardio session to pump up the intensity. Mix and match the drills any way you want.

Cone Slalom Set six to eight weight plates, dumbbells, or other small objects in a straight line about 1 yard apart. As fast as possible, run from one end of the line to the other, weaving back and forth between the objects, then turn and repeat, back to the starting point.

Speed Carioca Stand with your knees slightly bent and your arms extended out to your sides. Cross your left foot in front of your right foot to propel yourself to the right. Step to the right with your right foot and place your left foot behind it. (Rotate your hips as you move, but keep your eyes forward.) Continue cross-stepping as fast as possible for 5 to 15 yards, and then repeat to the left.

Ladder Run If you don't have a ladder, place several strips of tape or sticks on the ground about a foot apart. Quickly sidestep through the ladder, placing one foot in each box. Repeat in both directions. Add variety by lifting your knees high or keeping the motion extra low and fast. *Note:* You can do this without the ladder—just imagine it's there and go through the same high-stepping motions. But having markers will help prevent you from cheating.

Backpedal Sprint backward, keeping your eyes forward and maintaining a slight bend in your knees and hips. Use small, quick steps. Alternate backpedaling with forward sprints: Sprint 5 to 15 yards and backpedal back to the starting point.

Side Shuffle Push off with your left foot to propel yourself to the right. After your right foot lands, quickly step to the right with your left foot to bring your feet together. Continue for 5 to 15 yards, then reverse directions and shuffle back to the start.

Hexagon Jump These work for both plyometrics and agility. Set six sticks or strips of tape into a hexagon (or imagine one) and stand in the middle. Jump laterally to the right over each mark and back into the center as fast as you can, moving around the hexagon. You'll have to turn slightly to the left each time. Go around three times, then stop in the center and repeat to the left for three rotations.

Plateau Buster Add two more drills or add more intricate maneuvers. You can also combine the drills to make them harder or push yourself to sprint farther.

PLYOMETRIC TRAINING

Why you need it: To spike volleyballs, block basketballs, and yes, maybe even dunk. A recent study published in the *Journal of Athletic Training* verified that when done twice weekly, plyometrics improve vertical jump by nearly 6 percent. It turns out they can also elevate your strength training. Researchers at the College of New Jersey found that when subjects jumped before performing squats, they were able to handle 5 percent more weight. "Plyometrics excite the fast-twitch muscle fibers, the ones required for maximizing strength gains," explains study author Avery Faigenbaum, CSCS.

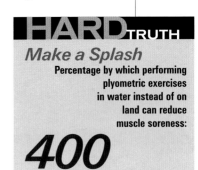

HARD TRUTH
Make a Splash
Percentage by which performing plyometric exercises in water instead of on land can reduce muscle soreness:

400

If you scored . . .

. . . less than 20 inches in the vertical jump:
Do 5 minutes of plyometric training two times a week. Pick two or three of the moves that follow and do two sets of the recommended repetitions.

. . . 20 inches or more in the vertical jump:
Aim for 10 minutes of plyometric training twice a week. Pick three or four of the moves below and do two or three sets of the recommended number of reps.

The Moves

Try incorporating plyometric drills into your warmup routine to maximize performance and strength gains. Make your movements quick, crisp, and explosive to, as Faigenbaum puts it, "turn on the nerves going to your muscles." Beginners, stay low: Keep movements close to the ground and progress slowly. Landing a high or deep jump could strain weak knees and ankles.

Skater Jump Balance on the ball of your left foot and jump as far as you can to the right. Land on your right foot and hold the landing for a second, then jump back to the left foot. Repeat 10 times.

Tuck Jump Stand with your feet shoulder-width apart and your knees slightly bent. Jump straight up as high as you can and bring your knees toward your chest. Land on the balls of your feet with your knees slightly bent. Do five jumps without pausing, and visualize that the next rebounding title is yours.

Step/Box Jump Stand with an exercise step in front of you. Jump forward onto the step with both feet and then jump down on the far side. Turn around and repeat five times. Next, jump laterally onto the step, land, and jump down on the opposite side. Then reverse. Do five repetitions in each direction. Keep your jumps quick and continuous, and progress until you're jumping onto a 12-inch-high box.

Two-Legged Bound Place five sticks or strips of tape about a yard apart in a straight line. Quickly jump as high and as far as you can over each marker. Repeat five times.

Squat-Jump Throw Stand with your feet shoulder-width apart, holding a medicine ball close to your chest. Bend your knees to lower your body about 6 inches, then jump as high as you can while pushing your arms straight up. Despite the name of the exercise, you never release the ball, so you can continue without stopping. Repeat five times.

Plyometric Pushup Assume the standard pushup position on an exercise mat. Lower yourself to the bottom position, then quickly push up with enough force so that your hands come off the floor. Catch yourself with your elbows slightly bent, then lower yourself with a controlled movement. Do 10 reps.

Plateau Buster Add another of the plyometric exercises or do more repetitions. Incorporate balance by turning two-legged jumps into one-legged versions (such as one-legged bounds).

BY MICHAEL MEJIA, CSCS

Make Your Workout Work Harder for You

How to design a regimen around your personal fitness goals

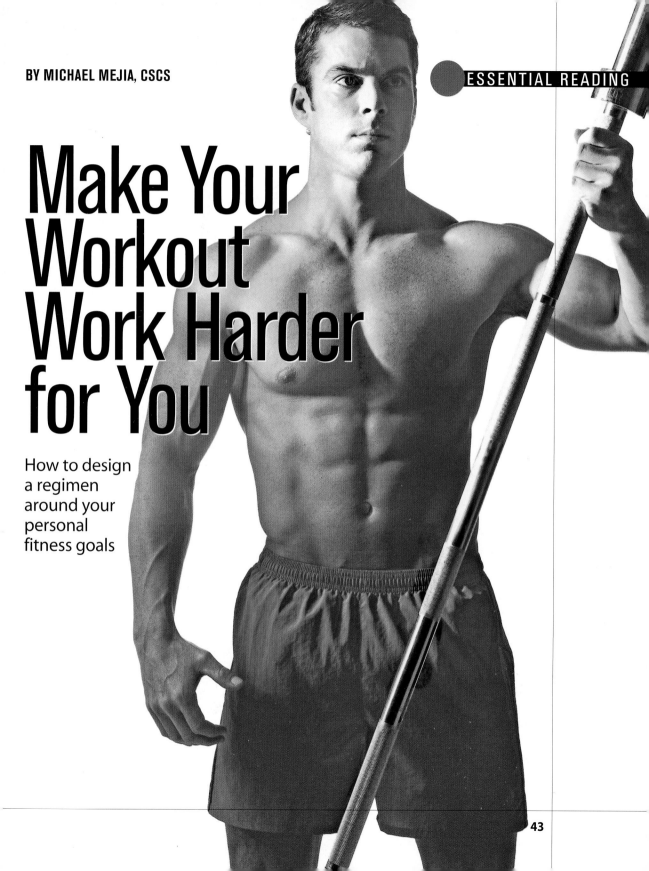

43

ere's a sign of the times: You can actually hire people to come to your house and organize your closets. They'll also do your garage, your attic, and the shed in your backyard. These people are tough on pack rats. They ask questions like "Why do you have this box of dog leashes, but no dog?"

My job isn't all that different. As a trainer, if I see something in a client's workout—or my own—that doesn't belong there, I get rid of it. If I see a redundant exercise, it's gone. Disorganized workout? I organize it. And if I see a client doing a program he got out of some old bodybuilding magazine, I throw the whole thing out and start over.

I can't come to your gym and fix your workout (or organize your closets). But I can tell you what you need to know to organize your own regimen, based on your goals, available time, and experience. I'll even throw in six sample workouts for beginner through advanced lifters.

Now, about those closets . . .

Goals

I assume the closet lady would start by asking, "What do you need this closet to do for you?" Me, I'd ask the same question, substituting the word "workout" for "closet." Usually, the answers fall into three categories.

Lose weight: If you're a beginner, start with a circuit routine in which you do 10 to 12 exercises one after the other, 10 to 15 repetitions per set, with little or no rest in between. Do two or three circuits.

If you're more advanced, try supersets: Do two exercises back-to-back, rest 60 sec-

Choose Your Workout
WEIGHT LOSS/OVERALL CONDITIONING

Do this workout if you're starting out and can exercise 2 days a week. Do the exercises as a circuit. Do 10 to 15 reps per set.

Leg press
Seated row
Squat (with light weight)
Dumbbell bench press
Leg curl
Shoulder press
Situp
Lat pulldown
Lunge
Back extension
Upright row

Do these workouts if you're experienced and can exercise 2 days a week. Do the exercises as supersets. Do 4 sets of 10 to 12 reps.

WORKOUT A
Barbell squat/seated row
Lunge/bench press

WORKOUT B
Deadlift/shoulder press
Pullup/weighted situp

If you're starting out and can exercise 3 days a week, do these workouts. Do them as straight sets. Do 8 to 12 reps per set, and rotate the workouts each week.

WORKOUT A
Leg press
Bench press
Lunge
Shoulder press
Situp

WORKOUT B
Deadlift
Lat pulldown
Leg curl
Single-arm row
Back extension

If you're experienced and can exercise 3 days a week, do these workouts. Do the exercises as supersets, and rotate the workouts each week.

WORKOUT A
Do 3 sets of 6 to 8 reps.
Bench press/dumbbell fly
Pullup/cable row
Shoulder press/lateral raise

WORKOUT B
Squat (5 sets of 5 reps)
Deadlift (5 sets of 5 reps)
Lunge (2 sets of 8 to 12 reps)
Leg curl (2 sets of 8 to 10 reps)
Standing calf raise (2 sets of 8 to 10 reps)

STRENGTH BUILDING

Do these workouts if you're starting out and can exercise 3 or more days a week. Do the exercises with heavy weights as straight sets: 5 sets of 5 repetitions.

WORKOUT A
Incline press
Squat
Dip
Barbell stepup

WORKOUT B
Single-leg deadlift
Chinup (or lat pulldown)
Leg curl
Seated row

WORKOUT C
Perform as supersets, 8 to 12 reps per set
Dumbbell bench press/leg press
Single-arm row/leg curl
Shoulder press/Swiss-ball crunch
Lat pulldown/back extension

Do these workouts if you're experienced and can exercise 4 days a week. Do the exercises as straight sets.

WORKOUT A (Strength)
Deadlift (8 sets of 3 reps)
Military press (8 sets of 3 reps)

WORKOUT B (Muscle Growth)
Bench press (3 sets of 8 reps)
Lunge (3 sets of 8 reps)
Bent-over row (3 sets of 8 reps)
Calf raise (3 sets of 8 reps)

WORKOUT C (Strength)
Squat (8 sets of 3 reps)
Weighted pullup

WORKOUT D (Muscle Growth)
Dumbbell shoulder press (3 sets of 8 reps)
Leg curl (3 sets of 8 reps)
Cable crunch (3 sets of 8 reps)
Dip (3 sets of 8 reps)

onds, and then repeat once or twice. There are many ways to do supersets, but for fat loss, I'd like to see you use as much muscle as possible. One way is to pair exercises that work completely different muscles, such as squats and seated rows.

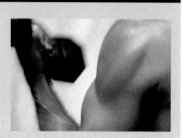
Build muscle: For most men, I recommend exercises that allow you to do 8 to 12 repetitions per set. You can do them as straight sets—complete a set, rest about 60 seconds, do the next set of the same thing, and keep going that way until you've finished all your sets and are ready to move on to the next exercise.

If you have more experience, try supersets, but not the way you did them for fat loss. Pair synergistic exercises—two moves that work the same muscles. Usually, the first is a compound move to work a lot of muscles, the second a single-joint exercise to focus on one large muscle. So barbell bench presses might be followed by dumbbell flies. Shoulder presses could lead in to lateral raises.

Gain strength: There's no secret here—heavy weights, low repetitions (usually three to five per set for the most important moves, such as squats, deadlifts, and bench presses), and longer rest (up to 4 minutes) between sets. You don't have to do every exercise this way, of course.

Start with low reps on your main moves, then do more repetitions with lighter weights and shorter rest periods on less important ones.

Available Time

This is akin to the closet lady saying, "What's your budget?" Before I design a program, I need to know how much time you're going to put in. I assume everyone is willing to work out 40 to 60 minutes per session. To me, that's a finite window, just as your closet is a finite size. If you want to do longer workouts, great—but if I can't give you a system that gets it done in an hour or less, there's something wrong with my program. The big variable here is how many days a week you're able and willing to work out.

Two days a week: No matter your level or goals, do total-body workouts. You want to hit your major muscles twice a week; otherwise, they'll be completely rested between workouts and will have no reason to grow.

If you're a beginner, stick to circuits, as I recommended above for fat loss. But if you're more interested in building muscle than in losing fat, I suggest doing sets of 8 to 12 reps, with perhaps a little more rest in between exercises.

Another option for saving time is to do antagonistic supersets. These pair up movements that involve opposite muscle actions, such as situps and back extensions.

Three days a week: If you're not a beginner, you can adopt a split routine. The easiest to remember is the upper-body/lower-body split. You alternate between them, so if you're training three times a week, you'll do upper-lower-upper 1 week, then lower-upper-lower the next. If you're working out four times a week, you'll do upper on Monday and Thursday, and lower on Tuesday and Friday.

What you do during those split routines depends on your goals (explained on pages 44 and 46) and your experience (explained below).

Experience

Beginners make gains with just about any type of program, so it's best to keep it simple and safe—fairly high repetitions, basic exercises, total-body workouts. The more experience you have, the more you'll benefit from heavier weights and lower repetitions, more advanced exercises and techniques, and split routines.

Another issue is recovery. A beginner can recover in 48 hours and do fine with three total-body workouts a week. A more advanced lifter needs to give his muscles more time to recover because he's hitting them harder.

Also, the more experienced you are, the less time you should spend on a program before moving on. A beginner can do the same program for 6 to 10 weeks without hitting a plateau. Grizzled iron vets may need to move on every 2 or 3 weeks. You probably fall somewhere in between.

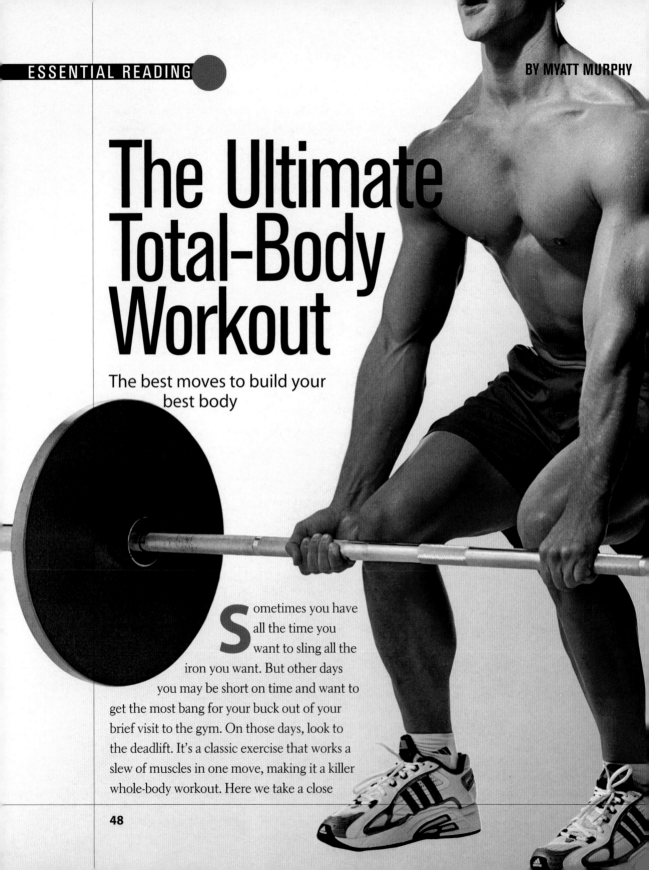

BY MYATT MURPHY

The Ultimate Total-Body Workout

The best moves to build your best body

Sometimes you have all the time you want to sling all the iron you want. But other days you may be short on time and want to get the most bang for your buck out of your brief visit to the gym. On those days, look to the deadlift. It's a classic exercise that works a slew of muscles in one move, making it a killer whole-body workout. Here we take a close look at the deadlift, and we throw in a few extra exercises just for good measure.

The Facts

Isolating muscle groups by using exercises that prevent other muscles from helping out can make the targeted muscles grow stronger and larger. But forcing your muscles to work with each other has tremendous benefits. Compound exercises like the deadlift, squat, and bench press allow you to handle heavier amounts of weight for even greater gains in strength—they work more than 85 percent of your body's muscles. Your legs, chest, and back are all primary muscle groups that require other, secondary muscle groups—the shoulders, triceps, biceps, abdominals, and

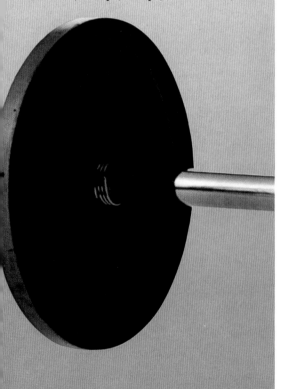

calves—to assist in every exercise. When it comes to a full-body workout, it's crucial to exhaust your primary muscles first and your secondary muscles last. The smartest order: legs first, upper body second, abs last.

The Payoff

A better body. Most total-body workouts use compound movements that require many muscles to work together. The end result is greater functional strength that can help improve your athletic performance and daily life.

Bigger muscles. Most compound exercises allow you to lift heavier amounts of weight than other exercises do. The more weight you're able to handle, the more your muscles are forced to grow.

A quicker workout. An exercise plan that targets every major muscle group in one session gives your body a complete workout in less time than a plan that focuses on each muscle group individually.

More power. Explosive movements such as jumping, sprinting, and throwing require all your muscles to work in cooperation. Creating that type of connection is easier when you perform exercises that leave your muscles no choice but to work together.

The Main Move

The deadlift is a simple, powerful exercise that adds size and strength from head to toe. Done correctly, the move requires many muscles—from your neck, back, and abdominals to your forearms, glutes, and quadriceps—to work together to lift the weight.

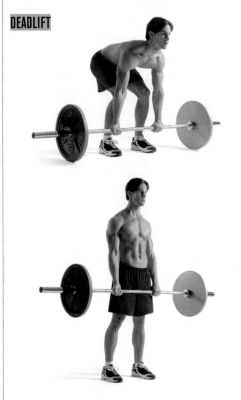

Stand straight with your feet shoulder-width apart and a light barbell on the floor in front of you, with the bar directly over your toes. Bend your knees and grasp the bar with an alternating grip (one palm facing you, the other facing away), your hands just outside your knees. Keeping your head and back straight, slowly stand, keeping the bar close to your body as you lift, until your legs are straight (knees unlocked). Pause, then slowly lower the bar to the floor.

Perfect Form

Head. Keep your head in line with your neck and back at all times. Tilting your head down to look at the bar places stress on your neck and trapezius muscles.

Arms. Keep your arms straight throughout the move. Don't shrug your shoulders or bend your elbows to help lift the weight.

Abs. Pull your abs in before you lift. This helps flatten your lower back for better support as you perform the move.

Lower back. Keep your back flat and in line with your head and neck. Arching your back redirects more effort onto your lower-back muscles, placing them at a greater risk of injury.

Butt. Squeeze your glutes at the start of the movement.

Hands. Space your hands shoulder-width apart and grab the bar using an alternating grip, which helps you keep it from slipping.

Knees. Avoid locking your knees as you straighten your legs at the top of the lift.

Legs. Begin to straighten your legs before you start to pull the weight from the floor so that there's tension in your arms. You should feel the bar comfortably sliding up and down your legs throughout the lift.

Feet. Your feet should be shoulder-width apart and flat on the floor at all times.

Mix and Max

Vary your stance. Instead of holding the bar with your hands shoulder-width apart, space them wider apart.

Change tools. Trade the barbell for a pair of dumbbells. You'll lift less weight, but having your arms down along your sides—palms facing in—can make it easier to balance as you go.

Adjust your approach. Instead of lifting the bar from the floor, place it on a squat rack or blocks so the bottoms of the weight plates are off the ground. This reduces the distance that you move the weight, allowing you to use heavier weights than usual.

The Workout

Multijoint exercises can give you the best full-body workout in the shortest time. These five exercises combine compound and functional moves so you'll work as many muscles as possible. After your deadlift routine, pick one exercise from section A (lower body), do the dumbbell bench press (section B, upper body), and pick one move from section C (abdominals). Then build your program using the chart below. You'll get a custom-made workout that will improve the strength, size, and performance of every muscle in your body—in less time than you would expect.

Get more: Stand with the top of your right foot resting on a weight bench. Slowly lower yourself into a lunge position. (Your right leg should be used only to help maintain your balance.) Press yourself back up and complete one set, then switch legs.

DUMBBELL LUNGE (A)

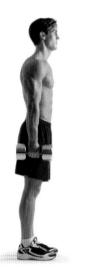
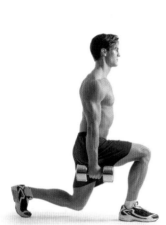

Stand holding a dumbbell in each hand, arms hanging at your sides, feet about 6 inches apart. Keeping your back straight, step forward with your right foot and lower your body until your right thigh is almost parallel to the floor. Push yourself back up to the starting position and repeat the move, this time stepping out with your left foot.

The Right Workout for You

Build the ultimate physique with our easy-to-use chart

YOUR LEVEL	WORK YOUR ENTIRE BODY	SETS OF EACH EXERCISE	REPETITIONS PER SET	SPEED OF EACH REP	REST BETWEEN SETS
Beginner	Three times a week	1–3	10–15	3–4 seconds up, 3–4 seconds down	30–60 seconds
Intermediate	Twice a week	2–4	8–12	2–3 seconds up, 2–3 seconds down	60–120 seconds
Advanced	Twice a week	3–5	6–8	2 seconds up, 2 seconds down	90–240 seconds

BARBELL SQUAT (A)

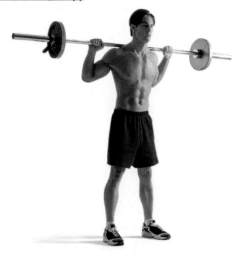

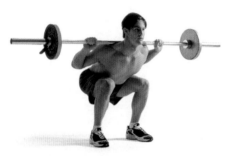

Place a barbell on a squat rack at about chest level. Grab the bar with an overhand grip slightly wider than shoulder-width apart, duck underneath it, and rest the bar across the backs of your shoulders. Lift the bar off the rack and step back. With your feet shoulder-width apart and your back straight, slowly squat until your thighs are almost parallel to the floor. Pause, then press yourself back up into a standing position.

Get more: Move your left foot forward so it's 2½ to 3 feet in front of your right foot. Squat until your left thigh is parallel to the floor, press yourself back up, and complete one set before repeating with your right foot in front of your left.

DUMBBELL BENCH PRESS (B)

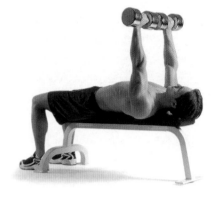

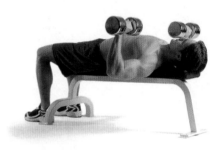

Grab a dumbbell in each hand (palms forward) and lie on a bench with your feet flat on the floor. Hold your arms straight above your chest. Slowly lower the weights to the sides of your chest. Pause, then press them back up.

Get more: Try doing the move one arm at a time. Start with both weights positioned by the sides of your chest, then slowly press one dumbbell above your chest while keeping the other in place. Lower the weight, then repeat the move with the other weight.

CROSS-KNEE TWISTING CRUNCH (C)

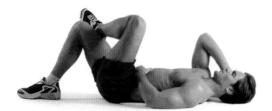

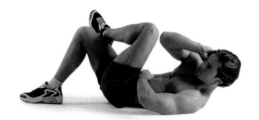

Lie on your back with your knees bent and your feet flat on the floor. Cross your left foot over your right knee. (Your left ankle should rest just below your right knee.) Place your right hand on the back of your head, pointing your elbow forward. (Your left hand can rest on your midsection.) Now, slowly curl your torso off the floor and twist to the left, drawing your right elbow to your left knee. Pause, then lower yourself back down and repeat. Finish the set, then switch leg positions to work the opposite side.

Get more: Straighten your legs and raise them so your feet are about 2 feet above the floor. As you curl your torso, simultaneously bend your knees toward your elbow; as you lower your torso, straighten your legs so your feet return to the starting position.

MEDICINE-BALL TWISTING CURL (C)

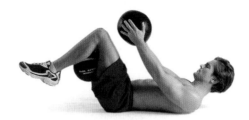

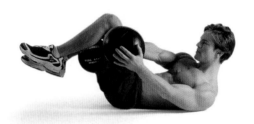

Lie on your back and place a small medicine ball under your knees. (Draw your feet toward your butt to pinch the ball in place.) Your thighs should be almost perpendicular to the floor. Hold another medicine ball with straight arms pointing at your thighs. Now slowly curl your head and shoulders off the floor and twist to the left. (The ball in your hands should end up at the outside of your left thigh.) Lower yourself, then repeat the move, this time twisting to the right.

Get more: Try holding the ball with your arms extended straight behind your head—your upper arms by your ears—at the start of the move. Then sweep the ball over your head and in front as you curl up and twist.

BY DAVID SCHIPPER

Make Your Cardio Count

Next time you race off to the gym, use these secrets for maximum effect

There's a Rube Goldberg aspect to cardiovascular-exercise machines. It's not all the levers and belts and pedals but the effort-to-reward ratio. Sometimes it seems we expend a lot of time, energy, and goofy-looking movement for too small a payoff. For all the hours we've spent on these gizmos, our pants should be looser. But maybe (as we've heard a few times in our lives) we're doing it all wrong.

Cardio machines are tremendous fat burners—when used correctly. And because you can work very hard in a very short time, they can make a lunchtime workout an exercise in efficiency or make a prework morning session not only possible but effective as well.

We asked the experts what they see people doing wrong on the leading machines and found out how we can squeeze more out of our time on them. Follow their suggestions and you'll burn more fat than the sweat-spraying cardio crazies with the blurry legs and burning lungs . . . and still have time for a smoothie afterward.

Rowing Machine

YOUR FORM

The mistake: Your hands bump your knees and "everything gets jumbled," says Mike Irwin, University of Pennsylvania lightweight varsity crew coach.

The fix: Think of the stroke as a dance, counting 1-2-3 and 3-2-1. On 1, push with your legs; on 2, "swing up" your body by leaning back; on 3, draw your arms to the bottom of your rib cage, spinning the flywheel. Then reverse it: 3, extend your arms; 2, swing your body forward from the hips; 1, bring your legs up after the handle passes your knees. "It should be a fluid motion when you tie it all together," says Irwin.

YOUR WORKOUT

The mistake: A long, steady slog. "You probably won't be able to maintain your power and form for the entire workout," Irwin says.

The fix: With medium resistance, do four to six 10-minute sets of rowing with 2 to 3 minutes of rest in between. "Your heart rate won't come all the way down, but

you'll be able to regroup and start fresh," says Irwin.

Treadmill

YOUR FORM

The mistake: Too much up and down and not enough levelheadedness, says Zack Barksdale, an exercise physiologist at the Cooper Aerobics Center in Dallas. You'll tire out your joints—and yourself—too soon.

The fix: Improve flexibility to smooth out your stride. Try leg swings—hold the handlebar, stand on one leg, and swing the other back and forth, keeping your upper body still. "It will loosen and warm you up, making your legs more pliable," says Barksdale.

YOUR WORKOUT

The mistake: Too many long, steady, flat runs.

The fix: Run shorter and harder, mixing speeds and inclines. You'll fatigue your muscles and your energy source more quickly, leading to more efficient fat burning throughout the day. Start with a 2 percent incline, and over several sessions work up to 10 percent. (Just walk at this point.) The more intense the workout, the shorter it can be.

Stationary Bike

YOUR FORM

The mistake: The seat is too low or too high. "It fatigues the legs a lot more if the seat is too low," says Brian Holdsworth, director of fitness at the Healthplex Sports Club in Indianapolis. A very low seat also adds stress on the knees. Set it too high and your hips rock from side to side, which is uncomfortable and inefficient, and it makes you look funny.

The fix: Adjust the seat, people! Sit on the seat and place your heel in the middle of the pedal, where the ball of your foot would normally go. You want your leg fully extended, straight down, at the lowest point of the pedal rotation. "When you move your foot to the correct position on the pedal, you'll have the right amount of bend," Holdsworth says.

YOUR WORKOUT

The mistake: Cruising instead of charging.

The fix: Vary the intensity, with 2 to 3 minutes of high-cadence pedaling and a 3-minute recovery, then repeat for 15 minutes. Stand occasionally. "Standing requires

Jump like a Champ

Why should you go out right now and buy a jump rope? Because 10 minutes of jumping rope can provide the same calorie burn as 30 minutes of running. Plus, when you get good, you'll look like a prize-fighter.

Rope jumping uses all your muscles and joints, says Buddy Lee, a jump-rope trainer and member of two US Olympic wrestling teams. It also requires some skill and practice. Here's some advice from Lee (go to buddyleejumpropes.com for more).

Balance: Your weight is on the balls of your feet, your knees slightly bent. Don't jump more than an inch. Keep your body upright, eyes front, and elbows close, and make small circles with your wrists.

The Jump: It's just a slight push, but it comes from the ankles, calves, knees, and hips. Push through the floor with the balls of your feet and point your toes downward as you lift off.

The Landing: Land softly by spreading the impact through your ankles, knees, and hips. Contact with the ground should be as brief as possible, your heels never touching the ground. Don't double bounce. That's too easy.

The Alternate Step: Jump with one foot. On the second turn of the rope, switch feet. Continue alternating feet (as if jogging in place) at a slow pace until you establish a comfortable rhythm. Lift your knees forward without kicking backward, which can cause your foot to catch on the rope.

The Program: With the basic bounce or alternate step, start with 10 sets of 10 jumps. Increase the number of jumps by 10 per set until you reach 100 nonstop. Gradually work toward 5 to 10 minutes of continuous jumping.

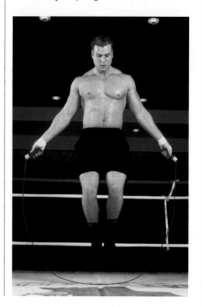

more muscle, not only to push the pedals, but also to support and balance your body," explains Joe Friel, author of *The Cyclist's Training Bible*.

Elliptical Trainer

YOUR FORM

The mistake: Too little resistance. "Some people go so fast that it's almost momentum working for them, as opposed to their having to propel the step," says Holdsworth.

The fix: Set the resistance correctly. Gliding isn't good. "When you make a revolution, you want to feel you're pushing the ramp down," says Holdsworth. "Have weight there rather than flipping around freely." As your balance improves, keep your hands at your sides; you'll recruit core muscles to keep yourself stable.

YOUR WORKOUT

The mistake: Falling into boring ruts.

The fix: Do intervals. "You'll be able to reach a higher intensity for a sustained period of time," says Holdsworth. Try 90-second blasts every few minutes, with recoveries twice as long. "As your fitness level increases, reduce the recovery time," says Holdsworth.

Stairclimber

YOUR FORM

The mistake: "People hold themselves up with their arms," says Holdsworth. Never put your arms straight down on the railing and lock your elbows. That's like using crutches.

The fix: Rest your hands on the bars only for balance. "The ideal movement is with your body upright, with just a slight lean forward," says Holdsworth, "as if you were leaning to walk up a flight of stairs but not bending over."

YOUR WORKOUT

The mistake: Too little resistance.

The fix: Go slower, with challenging resistance. "It'll make you work harder, your heart rate will be higher and faster, and you'll be able to maintain your time in the training zone longer," says Holdsworth. Result: You'll burn more fat.

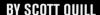

BY SCOTT QUILL

21 Ways to Stick with a Workout

Simple solutions for our favorite excuses

We hear you're ready for a gut-busting 2006. This is the year you'll stick to your muscle-building, fat-burning covenant: the New Year's resolution. No missed days. No empty calories. No wimp-outs. No excuses. No, really.

We believe you. More men join gyms in January than in any other month. Of the 16 percent of guys who resolve to work out more in the new year, however, 49 percent fail to adhere to their resolutions. We've heard all the excuses. (We've used a few ourselves.)

So we made a list of them—the

lame and the understandable. Then we called around to psychologists, dietitians, trainers, and men who manage to work out no matter how busy their lives are.

First, the legitimate excuses. We found four: You're sore; you're sick; you're exhausted; you're hurt. That's it.

Soreness means your body needs a break. "Recovery is as important as working out," says Carter Hays, CSCS, a Houston-based personal trainer. Overtraining keeps as many men from reaching their goals as undertraining does, says Hays. Illness means you should knock off and let your body fight the bug. If you're so tired you're drowsy, you could hurt yourself. And if you're injured—especially if you're experiencing joint pain—let your body heal.

As for the rest of the excuses, listen up.

"Looks like rain." *Men's Health* cover model Gregg Avedon lives in Florida. Do the names Charley, Frances, Ivan, and Jeanne mean anything to you? Avedon spent much of 2004 lifting storm shutters and storing away patio furniture, then taking cover. He still looks great. Avedon says your home gym—those dumbbells over there, and your chinup bar—makes staying in a viable option. You can also spice up your indoor cardio by jumping rope or running up and down stairs. Or tie both ends of a resistance band to a doorway, place a towel across your chest, face away from the door with the band (cushioned by the towel) across your chest, and run in place.

"I have no time." Combine things you do anyway—work, breathe—with athletics. Set up business meetings during which you walk or jog, play tennis with your date, take a spin class to find dates, or take your family hiking, suggests Charles Stuart Platkin, MPH, author of *The Automatic Diet*.

"I pack my gym bag and then *The O.C.* comes on." Get TiVo. Then tell yourself you're going to do just half of your regular routine. "It won't seem so insurmountable, and you'll end up doing the whole workout," says Edward Abramson, PhD, a clinical psychologist in Lafayette, California.

"I need my sleep." Pat Croce manages to stick with his workouts, and this father of two has been busy hosting his syndicated TV show, *Pat Croce: Moving In,* and opening a pirate museum in Key West, Florida. "Like me, you have to schedule fitness," he says. On the first of each month, Croce reviews

PEAK
performance

Work Out Longer

Next time you're having trouble finishing your indoor cardiovascular workout, don't blame it on the lack of scenery. Your body has a harder time staying cool indoors. What you need more than climate control is moving air—a breeze helps evaporate sweat to keep your body from overheating. It can work even better than having the air-conditioning cranked up during your workout, according to research. Evaporative cooling gives you more endurance, helping you run faster longer (or row, or step, or whatever the verb is that goes with the elliptical trainer). The solution: Get a big fan and point it at yourself. As long as we're not downwind.

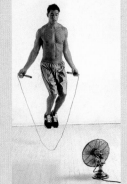

his schedule with his secretary and then his wife, and breaks it down into weeks. Every Sunday, he goes over the coming week, making sure there are gyms at hotels where he'll be staying.

"I don't want to spend $50 a month on a gym membership." Don't. January's the month to negotiate fees, trial months, or group discounts. Think you don't have the cash? Save $900 a year by switching from café mocha to metabolism-boosting green tea when you stop at Starbucks every morning.

"My gym sucks." So move. Changing gyms is an opportunity for you to upgrade your workout. See the next tip.

"I'm bored with my workout." "Throw it in reverse," says Gunnar Peterson, CSCS, author of *G-Force*. If you always do lat pulldowns with an overhand grip, switch to underhand. Do a reverse-grip bench press, reverse-grip curls, and reverse-grip triceps pushdowns. Do front squats, rear lunges, and dumbbell lateral raises with your palms up. Count backward, too, suggests Peterson. "It's like a blastoff—5, 4, 3, 2, 1, done."

"I never see results." Maybe you're not looking in the right places. Measure your waist, heart rate, and weight. Write them down. Then measure again after a week or two, says Croce. Celebrate even the smallest sign of progress. Muscles appear as fat melts.

"Four weeks, and no change in waistline, heart rate, or weight!" Whether you see results or not, you're strengthening your joints and connective tissues, which means you're laying a foundation for future muscle growth, says Peterson. Your diet, stress, sleep patterns, and other factors besides your workout may be holding you back, so don't give up.

"I have no energy." Eat. You need the fuel. "An active guy needs up to 1,000 calories more than an inactive guy," says Gay Riley, RD.

"I'm just making sure my body is getting adequate time to recover." After 72 hours of rest, you're just sliding backward. "But are you actually giving yourself a chance to recover?" asks Peterson. It's not all about time. Mix L-glutamine into your postworkout shake and eat a diet full of omega-3 fatty acids; they can assist with cellular reconstruction and the removal of metabolic wastes to help you recover faster, Peterson says.

"I always get hurt." This happens when you ratchet up your workout. Focus on losing 1 pound at a time or boosting your weights in 5-pound increments, says C.J. Murphy, MFS, owner of Total Performance Sports in Everett, Massachusetts. If you're used to doing 20 minutes on the treadmill, don't try a 2-hour road run. If you bench-press 50-pound dumbbells, don't go for 90.

Instead, make small increases in the difficulty of your workout, focus on form, and work with a spotter so you still have a safety net, Murphy says.

"My elbows/shins/pinkie toes hurt." "Pain is a sure sign something is awry with your exercise choices," says Murphy. This year, don't isolate body parts so much—your muscles should function as a team. If your shoulder hurts for a week after you do lateral raises, stop doing them. Find a variation that doesn't cause pain, he says.

"I don't want to look stupid trying to use those space-age machines." Approach new machines with enthusiasm. "That's a good way to broaden your fitness spectrum," says Peterson. Read the placard, ask a trainer for assistance, and give it a shot. Nobody's looking. "They're so into themselves that they're not even thinking about you," Peterson says.

"I'm bored again." Organize your workout differently for 1 to 2 weeks, says Peterson. Let's say you're usually a push-pull guy—you do chinups and leg curls one workout, bench presses and squats another. Try working antagonistic, or opposing, muscle groups, such as your back and chest. You can also change to an upper/lower split routine in which you alternate upper-body workouts with lower-body ones. Or try a total-body workout a few times a week.

"My buddy can't make it tonight." It's easy to blame others. "If you're serious about training, think of it like a job," says Murphy. "If your training partner was an employee who continually was late and had poor performance, what would you do? You'd fire him!"

"I hate working out alone." Go to the gym at the same time and on the same days. Say hi to people. You'll find others who are on your schedule, says Abramson.

"I should really stay with my wife tonight and help with the baby. Plus, *The O.C.* is on." Or you could help all three of you. More and more gyms have child-care centers so you and your wife can get away and spend time together—something that new parents need, says Abramson. Or go over the calendar with your wife: For every day she's out, you can schedule a workout.

"Everyone's going out for drinks." Join them once a week "and you won't appear standoffish," Abramson says. But eat first. By having your drinks with a meal, you won't drink, snack, and eat dinner later.

"But *The O.C.* is on!" "Create a commitment you can't get out of," says Platkin. Make an appointment with a trainer who will charge you whether you show or not.

"I commute for an hour. I'm not getting back in my car." Go straight from work twice a week, then work out at home the other nights. See "The Ultimate Total-Body Workout" on page 48 for a killer workout you can do while you watch *The O.C.*

Training Tips

ENERGY CRISIS

Q **I have a demanding job. How do I find the time and energy to get in shape?**

R.C., WICHITA, KANSAS

A Time's easy. Just pick an hour when you focus on something less important than your health. That's pretty much any hour, right? Use that time for exercise and reorganize your life around it. Energy takes care of itself once you start eating five or six small meals a day, cut out junk food and alcohol, and structure your life around that hour of exercise. You'll sleep better, feel better, shed fat, build muscle, and have *more* energy than ever before.

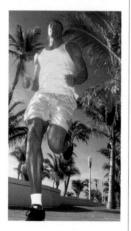

FIT FACT

No Need to See the Proof

Training helps, whether you can see it or not. Pennington Biomedical Research Center researchers studied 742 people on a 20-week training program and found that some improved in fitness, some lowered their risk of disease, and some got both benefits. "We haven't found anybody who does not respond at all for fitness or risk indicators," says study author Claude Bouchard, PhD.

SNOOZE OR LOSE

Q **If I've had only a few hours of sleep, should I force myself to go to the gym, or skip it?**

J.D., TEMPLE, TEXAS

A Take a pass. You don't need the added stress of a workout. Stress is cumulative—whether it's put on your body through training or by the demands of work and relationships. Remember, the goal of training should be to optimize health over a lifetime—elite bodies aren't built in a day. Manage your workouts based on long-term perspective, not short-term insecurity.

FREE YOURSELF

Q **I'm a relatively new lifter, and I use machines because I haven't been able to find a workout partner. What can I do to achieve better results?**

A.H., NEWTON, MASSACHUSETTS

A Work out with free weights, for starters. If you're worried about not having a spotter, use dumbbells for exercises like bench presses. Otherwise, you're kidding yourself if you think you can pack on significant muscle mass using machines. The best muscle builders you can do are squats and deadlifts, and no machine we've seen truly simulates these exercises.

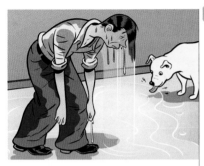

What's the fastest way to stop sweating after a workout?

P.O., MIAMI BEACH, FLORIDA

A cold shower works wonders, but it also stinks. The only way to avoid massive trickle stains after your lunchtime workout or, even worse, as you get ready for a date is to lower your exercise-elevated core body temperature. Eric Durak, MSc, president of Medical Health and Fitness in Santa Barbara, California, suggests running your wrists under cold water for a minute or two. This helps cool the blood that's close to the skin's surface. The blood circulates through your body and, voilà, you no longer need to sweat. Dipping your feet in a pool or lake works, too. (So does jumping in.)

Is it bad to work out with sore muscles?

T.F., DERBY, KANSAS

Soreness can be a normal workout side effect—or a sign that you have an injury. A good lifting session "hurts" muscles—they're slightly torn, so they can regrow bigger and stronger. If it's the kind of soreness you usually feel, go ahead and work out. Just take it easy so you don't injure muscles before they can recover. But if it's a new, localized pain, back off until it goes away.

Is it okay to do pushups and situps at home on days when I don't lift at the gym?

J.J., ST. PAUL, MINNEAPOLIS

It's fine, if you don't mind slouching shoulders and a predisposition to injury. The pushup is a great exercise, but the chest and abs are commonly overworked. Focus on regeneration exercises—moves that help your recovery, such as bridges for your core and Swiss-ball Ys (lie facedown on a Swiss ball and raise your arms—thumbs up—forward and out so your body forms a Y) for your rotator cuffs. When you get back to the gym, you'll be an all-star—and you'll avoid winding up on the DL.

The Eyes Have It

Who could have seen this coming? Your eyes benefit from strength training. Researchers at Mississippi State University report that you can reduce your risk of glaucoma with bench presses. In the study, 30 people who performed three sets of leg presses or bench presses reduced the pressure within their eyes, called intraocular pressure (IOP), by 13 percent and 15 percent, respectively. "Anything that lowers IOP reduces the pressure on the optic nerve, thus reducing the likelihood of nerve damage and glaucoma," says Joseph Chromiak, PhD, the lead study author. Exercises that recruit a lot of muscle mass, such as bench presses or squats, reduce pressure best, Chromiak says.

BUILD BIG MUSCLES

We're big thinkers at *Men's Health*. Meaning, we think that if a guy takes the time to hit the gym, then his muscles should be big to show for it.

You need to think big, too. If you sling iron the right way, you don't have to take off your shirt to reveal big muscles. They ripple through your T.

And since looking more ripped is the goal of 70 percent of guys who work out, we filled the following pages with big ideas to help you get there. With the shortcuts, workouts, and training tips in this section, you'll be busting out of your Hanes faster than the Hulk. So whether you're looking to build a better body for yourself or to turn some heads, we say build it and whatever you're after will come.

BY SCOTT QUILL

Train like an Animal

Attack this preworkout routine to unleash your muscular potential

A cheetah doesn't need much of a warmup. A leg stretch, a back arch, a yawn; then it's time to scare up some dinner—not a problem when your top speed is nearly 70 miles an hour.

We humans can't get away with that. We need to warm up before exerting ourselves. So what do we do before a gym workout? We jog, we swing our arms in little circles, and we declare ourselves ready.

It's time to evolve. If you lift hard, play hard, or want to boost your training to a new level, start with your warmup.

What follows is a preworkout routine inspired by nature's beasts. Mark Verstegen, MS, CSCS, calls this an "active and dynamic warmup," meaning it does everything you need for a strong workout. Verstegen is the author of *Core Performance* and owner of Athletes' Performance in Tempe, Arizona, and Carson, California. So he's seen his share of arm circles—which are okay; they're just not enough.

This warmup will elevate your heart rate and your core temperature—basics that too many men ignore. More important, it will activate the muscle groups you'll need in your lifting and will increase bloodflow to them.

The best part: This warmup will make you strong. That's because you'll be applying stress to your muscles in stretched positions and you'll be moving in several directions. It will also create great long-term flexibility in just 2 weeks by actively elongating and contracting your muscles through new ranges of motion.

What's the investment? About 7 to 10 minutes in addition to any traditional static stretches (stretch and hold) and foam-roll exercises you do. The benefit? A stronger, more athletic, more injury-resistant body.

This list draws from animals ranging from the lowly inchworm to the mighty, uh, donkey. Not that we can't learn from cheetahs. They have semiretractable claws for traction—we could stand to change our running shoes every 300 to 500 miles or so. We can't match a cheetah's 20-foot stride, but we can lengthen ours by running uphill and increase the frequency of our strides by running downhill.

You can still do your arm circles. But from now on, think outside the cage, and get warm.

THE INCHWORM

The inchworm is stable on any surface. This exercise, also known as the hand walk, stretches your hamstrings, calves, glutes, and lower back—"crucial for you to build a stable platform to operate on," says Robert Dos Remedios, CSCS, director of speed, strength, and conditioning at College of the Canyons in Santa Clarita, California.

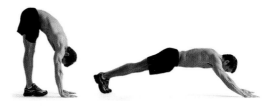

Stand with your legs straight and your hands on the floor. (You'll probably need to begin with your hands a couple of feet in front of you.) Keeping your legs straight, walk your hands forward as far as possible. Hold for 3 to 5 seconds. Then take tiny steps to walk your feet back to your hands. Hold again for 3 to 5 seconds. Repeat for a set of five.

THE SCORPION

This nasty arthropod has eight legs, a 12-pack, and poison. Get your edge by stretching your hip flexors, quadriceps, and abs, says Jon Crosby, CSCS, performance director at Velocity Sports Performance in Baltimore.

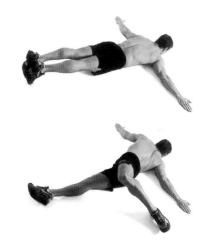

Lie on your stomach with your arms straight out at your sides and your legs straight, so your body forms a T. Keeping your arms still, thrust your left heel toward your right hand by squeezing your glutes (your butt) and bending your knee. Bring your leg back to the starting position, then try to touch your right heel to your left hand. Do five reps with each leg.

THE COBRA

A cobra has a cool expandable neck hood to intimidate enemies. This Swiss-ball cobra stretches your intimidation muscles—pecs, biceps, and front deltoids. It also strengthens your rhomboids, rear deltoids, lower trapezius, and triceps.

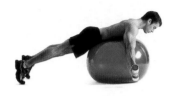

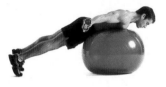

Lie facedown on a Swiss ball with your abs drawn in and your arms hanging down, holding light dumbbells. Raise your arms straight back until they're in line with your body, and pull your shoulder blades down and together. Hold the stretch for 2 to 3 seconds, then return to the starting position and repeat 10 times.

THE FROG

Jump squats are a way of life for amphibians. For you to build powerful legs, it's crucial to loosen the joints of your lower body, especially your hips. Tight hips hinder your ability to squat, says Crosby. What's more, when the piriformis—a muscle that attaches to your hip—gets tight, it yanks on your lower back, causing back pain, Crosby says. The frog thrust stretches and strengthens the hips, lower back, and groin muscles.

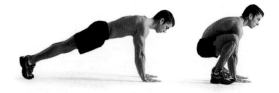

Assume the pushup position. With your hands under your shoulders and your abs drawn in, punch your knees to your chest so that your feet land in between your elbows, then push your legs back to the starting position. When you're comfortable with this, punch your knees forward so that they land by your hands and outside your elbows. (This is the frog thrust.) Then kick your legs back to the starting position. Do one set of five repetitions.

THE DONKEY

Any jackass can handle this move, which strengthens your hamstrings, hips, and glutes, according to Dos Remedios.

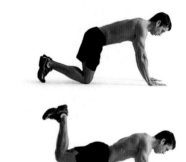

Get down on your hands and knees and kick your left leg back and up as high as you can. Keep your knee bent at a 90-degree angle and your back flat. (Don't hyperextend your back.) Finish by pulling your knee to your chest to stretch your glutes and lower back. Do a set of 10 to 15 reps, then repeat on the other side.

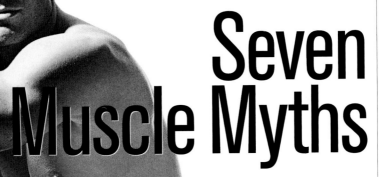
BY SCOTT QUILL

Seven Muscle Myths

We iron out what's true and what's not

The guy lifting beside you looks like he should write the book on muscle. Talks like it, too. He's worked out since the seventh grade, he played D-1 football, and he's big. But that doesn't mean he knows what he's talking about. Starting now, ignore him.

The gym is infested with bad information. Lies that start with well-intentioned gym teachers trickle down to students who become coaches, trainers, or know-it-all gym-rat preachers. Lies morph into myths that endure because we don't ask questions, for fear of looking stupid.

Scientists, on the other hand, gladly look stupid—that's why they're so darn smart. Plus, they have cool human-performance laboratories where they can prove or disprove theories and myths. Here's what top exercise scientists and expert trainers have to say about the crap that's passed around in gyms. Listen up and learn. Then go ahead—question it.

Myth #1

Lifting incredibly slowly builds incredibly big muscles. Lifting superslowly produces superlong workouts—and that's it. University of Alabama researchers recently studied two groups of lifters doing a 29-minute workout. One group performed exercises using a 5-second up phase and a 10-second down phase; the other, a more traditional approach of 1 second up and 1 second down. The faster group burned 71 percent more calories and lifted 250 percent more weight than the superslow lifters did.

The real expert says: "The best increases in strength are achieved by doing the up phase as rapidly as possible," says Gary Hunter, PhD, CSCS, the lead study author. "Lower the weight more slowly and under control." There's greater potential for growth during the lowering phase, and when you lower with control, there's less chance of injury.

Myth #2

If you eat more protein, you'll build more muscle. To a point, sure. But put down the shake for a sec. Protein promotes the muscle-building process, called protein synthesis, "but you don't need exorbitant amounts to do this," says John Ivy, PhD, coauthor of *Nutrient Timing*. If you're working out hard, consuming more than 0.9 to 1.25 grams of protein per pound of body weight is a waste. Excess protein breaks

PEAK
performance

Worth the Wait

Just wait—your bench press will improve. University of Kansas researchers studied 28 men performing sets of bench presses to failure. The men who rested for at least 3 minutes between sets performed 32 percent better in the second set than did those who rested for only a minute. "When muscle fatigues, the concentration of hydrogen ions in the muscle rises, which can make it harder to produce force," says Michael Godard, PhD, the senior study author and director of the university's applied-physiology laboratory.

A second study published in the *Journal of Sports Medicine and Physical Fitness* confirms that longer rest periods lead to greater gains in strength. Researchers had men do leg extensions twice a week for 6 weeks. The men who rested for 160 seconds between sets generated twice as much force with their quadriceps as those who rested for only 40 seconds. Lead study author Danny Pincivero, PhD, says the longer rest periods allow your muscles to recover so you can activate the maximum amount of force in subsequent sets.

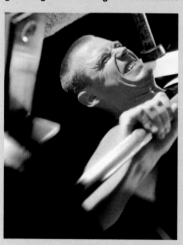

down into amino acids and nitrogen, which are either excreted or converted into carbohydrates and stored.

The real expert says: More important is *when* you consume protein and that you have the right balance of carbohydrates with it. Have a postworkout shake of three parts carbohydrates and one part protein. Eat a meal several hours later, and then reverse that ratio in your snack after another few hours. "This will keep protein synthesis going by maintaining high amino acid concentrations in the blood," says Ivy.

Myth #3

Leg extensions are safer for your knees than squats are. And cotton swabs are dangerous when you push them too far into your ears. It's a matter of knowing what you're doing. A recent study in *Medicine & Science in Sports & Exercise* found that "open-chain" exercises (those in which a single joint is activated, such as the leg extension) are potentially more dangerous than closed-chain moves (those that engage multiple joints, such as the squat and the leg press). The study found that leg extensions activate your quadriceps muscles slightly independently of each other, and just a 5-millisecond difference in activation causes uneven compression between the patella (kneecap) and thighbone, says Anki Stensdotter, the lead study author.

The real expert says: "The knee joint is controlled by the quadriceps and the hamstrings. Balanced muscle activity keeps the patella in place and appears to be more

easily attained in closed-chain exercises," says Stensdotter. To squat safely, hold your back as upright as possible and lower your body until your thighs are parallel to the floor (or at least as far as you can go without discomfort in your knees). Try front squats if you find yourself leaning forward. Although it's a more advanced move, the weight rests on the fronts of your shoulders, helping to keep your back upright, Stensdotter says.

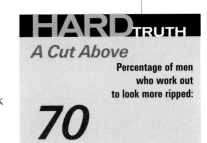

Myth #4

Never exercise a sore muscle. Before you skip that workout, determine how sore you really are. "If your muscle is sore to the touch or the soreness limits your range of motion, it's best that you give the muscle at least another day of rest," says Alan Mikesky, PhD, director of the human performance and biomechanics laboratory at Indiana University–Purdue University at Indianapolis. In less severe instances, an "active rest" involving light aerobic activity and stretching, and even light lifting, can help alleviate some of the soreness. "Light activity stimulates bloodflow through the muscles, which removes waste products to help in the repair process," says David Docherty, PhD, a professor of exercise science at the University of Victoria in Canada.

The real expert says: If you're not sore to the touch and you have your full range of motion, go to the gym. Start with 10 minutes of cycling, then exercise the achy muscle by performing no more than three sets of 10 to 15 repetitions using a weight that's no heavier than 30 percent of your one-rep maximum, says Docherty.

Myth #5

Stretching prevents injuries. Maybe if you're a figure skater. Researchers at the Centers for Disease Control and Prevention reviewed more than 350 studies and articles examining the relationship between stretching and injuries and concluded that stretching during a warmup has little effect on injury prevention. "Stretching increases flexibility, but most injuries occur within the normal range of motion," says Julie Gilchrist, MD, one of the study's researchers. "Stretching and warming up have just gone together for decades. It's simply what's done, and it hasn't been approached through rigorous science."

The real expert says: Warming up is what prevents injury, by slowly increasing your

How Strong Are You?

The truth is trickier than you think

When exercise experts look at strength, they look beyond the bench press and squat, which measure only absolute strength—the amount of force you can exert. But a bench-pressing behemoth with an injured shoulder is not strong. "The essence of strength is being able to use the right muscle at the right time with the right amount of force to accomplish your goal," says Mike Clark, MS, CSCS, president of the National Academy of Sports Medicine.

His definition of a strong man: a guy who can perform any exercise or daily task without pain or injury. This starts with understanding that your muscular system comprises two systems, one for movement and one for stabilization. The movement system produces force by using big muscles like your pecs and lats. The stabilizing system controls your joints and utilizes smaller muscles like your lower trapezius, your posterior deltoids, and the muscles of the rotator cuff.

"Most injuries occur because the stabilization system is not strong and the movement system is overly dominant," says Clark. You need to build both equally to avoid injury and perform better.

Alternate strength and stabilization exercises to enhance your endurance. For instance, do Swiss-ball pushups immediately after you bench-press; perform a squat followed immediately by a single-leg squat. If your stabilizing muscles are obviously weak— your shoulders are rounded, for instance—then begin your workouts with stabilizing exercises.

Aim to improve posture, flexibility, and power as well. You can follow strength exercises with power moves such as the medicine-ball chest pass, plyometric pushup, and jump squat. Incorporate core and flexibility moves (see "The Five Pillars of Fitness" on page 32) to round out your routine.

bloodflow and giving your muscles a chance to prepare for the upcoming activity. To this end, Dr. Gilchrist suggests a thorough warmup, as well as conditioning for your particular sport. Of course, flexibility is a good thing. If you need to increase yours so it's in the normal range (touching your toes without bending your knees, for instance), do your stretching when your muscles are already warm.

Myth #6

You need a Swiss ball to build a stronger chest and shoulders. Don't abandon your trusty bench for exercises like the chest press and shoulder press if your goal is strength and size. "The reason people are using the ball and getting gains is because they're weak as kittens to begin with," says Craig Ballantyne, CSCS, owner of turbulencetraining.com. You have to reduce the weight in order to press on a Swiss ball, so you get less out of the exercise, he says.

The real expert says: A Swiss ball is great for variety, but center your chest and shoulder routines on exercises that are performed on a stable surface, Ballantyne says. Then use the ball to work your abs.

Myth #7

Always work out with free weights. Sometimes machines can build muscle better—for instance, when you need to isolate specific muscles after an injury or when you're too inexperienced to perform a free-weight exercise. If you can't complete a pullup, you won't build your back muscles. Do lat pulldowns to develop strength in this range of motion, says Greg Haff, PhD, director of the strength research laboratory at Midwestern State University in Wichita Falls, Texas.

The real expert says: "Initially, novice athletes will see benefits with either machines or free weights, but as you become more trained, free weights should make up the major portion of your training program," says Haff. Free-weight exercises mimic athletic moves and generally activate more muscle mass. If you're a seasoned lifter, free weights are your best tools to build strength or burn fat.

Double Your Muscle

Partner up and reach your workout goals faster with these six moves

BY MARK VERSTEGEN, MS, CSCS

How did the Red Sox's Jason Varitek become such a threat on the ball field? Talent, to be sure, but only in tandem with a wicked-hard work ethic. I know, because I've seen him in action—not just behind the plate but at Athletes' Performance, my training facility in Tempe, Arizona. Jason and some of his teammates work out there during the off-season to build the strength they'll need for a 162-game schedule, plus several more games in October.

These pros push each other. You should try it, too. A training partner can motivate you, challenge you, and hold you accountable.

- Men who train with a partner bench-press more than those who train alone, according to research from Arizona State University.

- A training partner can watch and correct your form to help protect you from injury.

- Friendly competition keeps workouts fresh and pushes you to elevate your game.

- The pressure to be there for a teammate makes you less likely to skip out on a workout.

First, you need a partner. Approach a friend, co-worker, or fellow gym member and propose a realistic training schedule. Even if you can fit in only a couple of sessions a week, it'll be enough to build the partnership and encourage you to work harder on the other days.

Once you're armed with an extra pair of biceps, incorporate the following partner-assisted exercises into your training routine or perform them as a full-body workout. Consider it spring training for an all-star body.

SEATED MEDICINE-BALL THROW

You lie faceup on the floor with your back flat and knees bent, holding a 6-pound medicine ball. Extend your arms beyond your head so the ball is just above the floor.

Your partner sits 5 to 10 feet in front of you with his feet flat on the floor, knees bent, and arms straight overhead so he's ready to catch your pass.

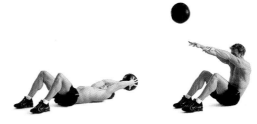

The move. Keeping your arms straight, curl your body up and throw the ball to your partner's hands. Remain in the sitting position. After he catches the ball, he should slowly lower himself to the floor, then explosively throw the ball back to you. Keep your feet planted at all times as you toss the ball back and forth. Aim for two or three sets of 8 to 20 repetitions.

Get better. As this becomes easy, add repetitions and sets, use a heavier medicine ball, or sit on a Swiss ball or the front edge of a Bosu Balance Trainer.

SEATED MEDICINE-BALL ROTATION

You sit on the floor with your knees bent and feet flat, and lean back (chest up, stomach tight, spine straight) at a 45-degree angle from the floor. Maintain this angle throughout.

Your partner stands on your toes, holding a medicine ball.

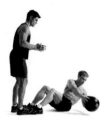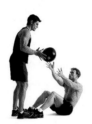

The move. Have your partner lob the ball toward the outside of your left hip. Catch the ball with your arms straight, and rotate your torso to the left to nearly touch the ball to the floor. Quickly reverse the motion to throw the ball back to your partner, who should catch it and throw it to your right side. Rotate from side to side with your shoulders, not just your arms. Try two or three sets of 8 to 20 repetitions.

BACK-EXTENSION THROW

You lie across a 45-degree hyperextension bench, tucking your ankles securely under the footpads. Your thighs should lie flat against the pad in front, leaving you enough room to bend at the waist without restriction. Keep your knees unlocked.

Your partner stands a few feet away with a 6-pound medicine ball.

The move. Have your partner throw the medicine ball just above your head. Catch it

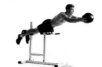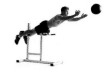

and slowly lower yourself with perfect posture until you feel a stretch in your hamstrings. Then explosively contract your glutes, hamstrings, and arms to throw the ball underhand back to your partner. Repeat for two or three sets of 6 to 12 repetitions.

EZ-CURL-BAR BICEPS CHALLENGE

You set up an EZ-curl bar or barbell with a weight that challenges both you and your training partner.

Your partner stands facing you.

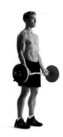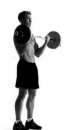

The move. Perform a set of 10 curls in a 3-0-1 tempo (3 seconds down, no rest, 1 second up). Then, instead of setting the bar down, hand it to your partner so he can do 10 repetitions. Hand it back and forth for nine reps, then eight, and so on. Work your way down until you've each done a single repetition with the bar, then place it on the floor, rest for 30 seconds, and try another set. Work up to three sets of this routine.

KNEELING HAMSTRING CURL

You kneel on a folded towel or a stack of three exercise mats, with your toes pulled toward your shins. Keep your hands in front of your chest.

Your partner sits behind you, facing your back, pressing down on your lower legs with his hands.

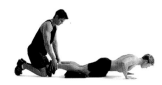

The move. Keep your abs tight, chest up, and hips forward so your body forms a straight line from your ears to your knees. Maintain this posture as you lower your torso toward the floor, while resisting gravity with your hamstrings and calves. Control the range of motion as far as you can, catch yourself with your hands, then push off the floor to assist your hamstrings and glutes in pulling you back up to the starting position. Repeat for two or three sets of 3 to 10 repetitions.

Get better. When you've mastered this, do it like Varitek: He holds a 25-pound plate on his chest, touches his chest to the floor, then pulls himself back up for three sets of six to eight repetitions.

LEG CIRCUIT RACE

You race against the clock and your partner to pump up your legs. Stand with your feet shoulder-width apart.

Your partner stands off to the side and waits for his turn.

The move. Start by doing 20 body-weight squats, lowering your body until your thighs are parallel to the floor, at a rate of one squat per second. Next, perform 10 forward lunges with each leg, then 10 lunges to the side with each leg. (Again, aim for one rep per second.) Finally, do 10 squat jumps—push off explosively so your feet leave the floor at the top of the move.

Try to complete this routine in 75 seconds. Do one to three sets, either head-to-head with your partner or alternating sets to see who's more fit.

Cheaters Prosper

Master perfect form, then learn some safe, smart shortcuts

Cheating is natural, and cheating works. Not WorldCom cheating, not she'll-never-find-out cheating, but gym cheating. Do a quick scan: You'll see plenty of guys taking form shortcuts to lift heavier weights. And their biceps seem to be getting bigger by the minute.

The standard line from trainers is that you'll get better results by using correct form, even if you have to lighten the load. That's because performing an exercise the way it's designed guarantees you're moving the weight with the intended target muscles. But results don't lie.

You can cheat your way to more muscle by using momentum, shorter ranges of motion, and body English. In fact, it's your natural instinct because it makes heavy weights easier to lift. You're still using the intended target muscles; you're just giving them a little help.

The problem is that cheating can be dangerous. Trying to lift as much weight as you can, any way you can, puts the stability of your

BY SCOTT QUILL

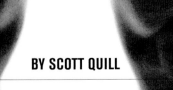

spine and joints at risk. And that increases the chance of tearing muscles, tendons, and ligaments. Or losing control of an overloaded barbell in an undesirable position, such as above your neck.

You can, however, cheat the smart way. But first you must master perfect form so you'll develop the muscle control needed to cheat safely and effectively. Follow our guide to learn the right and wrong ways to perform both the standard and "cheat" versions of five classic moves.

The Bench Press

The typical cheat: Bouncing a heavy barbell off your chest to help lift it back to the starting position.

Why it's dumb: It could kill you. "This may be the riskiest thing men do in the gym," says Craig Ballantyne, CSCS, owner of turbulencetraining.com. Bouncing the bar can lead to a loss of control, putting you at risk of a crushed neck and asphyxiation.

How to perfect your form: Before you bench, put a rolled-up towel down the middle of your upper body so that one end is at the center of your chest. Aim for the end of the towel on each repetition. Concentrating on accuracy ensures that you'll have control of the weight, says Ballantyne.

How to cheat smart: Try this touch-and-go "towel press." Use 50 percent of the weight that you usually use for six to eight repetitions. Do eight sets of three repetitions with 30 seconds' rest after each set. Place the towel on your chest and lower the bar as quickly as you can; as soon as the bar

touches the towel, push it up as fast as possible. Imagine that if the bar touches the towel for too long, it'll burn your chest.

The benefit: You'll learn to lift fast under control, which will translate into greater strength when you do a normal bench-press workout, Ballantyne says.

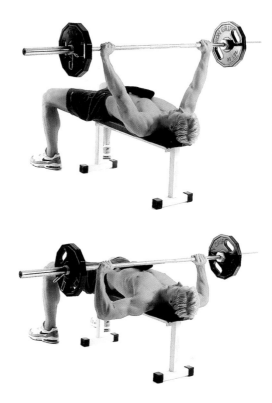

The Squat

The typical cheat: Doing the "lazy man's squat"—that is, reversing the movement before your thighs are parallel to the floor.

Why it's dumb: It increases your risk of knee injury. University of Auburn researchers found that the most unstable knee angle is 90 degrees—when your upper thighs are about 2 inches above parallel to the floor.

How to perfect your form: Lower yourself until the backs of your thighs touch your calves, says Alwyn Cosgrove, CSCS, owner of Results Fitness in Santa Clarita, California.

How to cheat smart: Use the "quarter squat" to supersize lagging quadriceps. Choose a weight that's about 20 percent more than you'd normally use for a full squat, and lower your body about 6 inches—until your knees are bent 60 degrees—pause, then return to the starting position.

The benefit: The quarter squat allows you to use heavier weights on your quadriceps while limiting the involvement of your hamstrings and calves. And it's safe because you reverse the movement well before your knees reach the 90-degree point.

The Biceps Curl

The typical cheat: Leaning back to curl a heavy weight.

Why it's dumb: It transfers the load unevenly from the front of your body to the back, and that can damage the muscles, ligaments, and joints of your back.

How to perfect your form: Stand against a wall when you curl, or hold a Swiss ball against the wall with your back, says Cosgrove. To practice even stricter form, keep your elbows in contact with the wall or ball for the entire lift.

How to cheat smart: Try this version of the "cheat curl." Hold a pair of heavy dumbbells at arm's length at your sides, palms

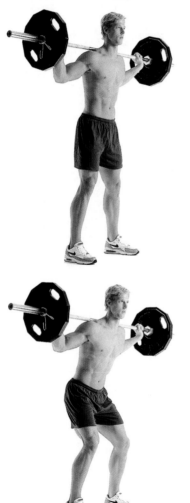

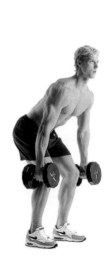

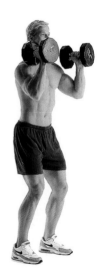

facing each other. Keeping your back naturally arched, lean forward at your hips and bend your legs until the dumbbells are next to your knees. Curl the dumbbells, push your hips forward, and straighten your legs all at the same time, until you're standing upright and the dumbbells are almost resting on your shoulders.

The benefit: You'll curl heavy weights without hurting your back. For an even greater muscle-building effect, lower the dumbbells as slowly as you can.

The Lat Pulldown

The typical cheat: Leaning back while pulling the bar down, using body weight and momentum to move the weight.

Why it's dumb: It reduces the focus on the target muscle—the latissimus dorsi—and increases the risk of injury to your lower and upper back, says Scott Rankin, CSCS, a strength coach in Toronto.

How to perfect your form: Think pullup, not pulldown. Keep your body upright throughout the move. Imagine you're pulling your chest to the bar instead of the bar to your chest. Or try this move: Sit upright on a Swiss ball and pull the bar straight down to your chest as you squeeze your shoulder blades together. If you try to use momentum to pull the bar down, you'll fall off the ball, says Rankin.

How to cheat smart: Do the "incline pulldown." Grab the lat-pulldown bar with a shoulder-width, overhand grip and lean back at your hips (keeping your back naturally arched) until your torso is at a 45-degree angle from the floor. Without moving your upper body, pull the bar down to the tops of your shoulders.

The benefit: It works the often neglected upper-back and rear-deltoid muscles.

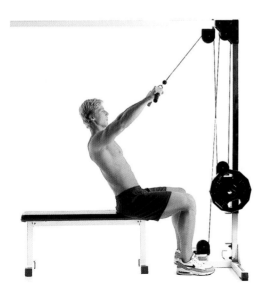
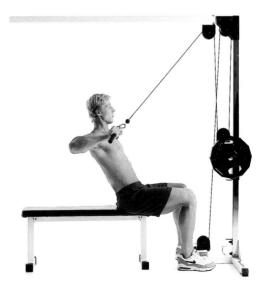

The Hanging Knee Raise

The typical cheat: Raising your knees to your chest without curling your torso, which is the key to working your abdominal muscles, says John Williams, CSCS, co-owner of Spectrum Conditioning in Port Washington, New York.

Why it's dumb: It makes the focus of the exercise your hip flexors, not your abs.

How to perfect your form: Grab a pullup bar with a shoulder-width, overhand grip and hang from the bar with your knees slightly bent and feet together. Imagine that you have no legs, and tilt your pelvis as high as you can by pulling your hips up and in. Aim for your knees to touch your shoulders.

The Replacements

Look weak to grow strong

You don't always need to use big weights to produce big results. These ego-crushing moves from Michael Mejia, CSCS, *Men's Health* contributing editor, force even the strongest men to use minimal weight. Substitute them for the standards for 3 weeks, then switch back to measure your gains. Be prepared: You'll even impress yourself.

King Squat (Instead of Squat)

Works quadriceps, abdominals, lower back. It makes your quadriceps work more while decreasing the involvement of your hips.

Place a barbell (with no added weight) on your upper back and set your feet shoulder-width apart. Without moving your legs or upper body, push your hips forward. This will "flatten" your back so that your spine is in a neutral position instead of naturally curved. Lower your body as far as you can without allowing your back to round or arch. Don't worry if you're not able to lower your thighs to at least parallel to the floor—most guys can't. Since the weight's light, the stress on your knees is minimized.

Reverse Pushup with Elbows Out (Instead of Lat Pulldown)

Works rhomboids, rear deltoids, trapezius. This variation deemphasizes your latissimus dorsi muscle, which dominates the movement when your elbows are closer to your sides.

Secure a bar 3 to 4 feet above the floor (in a power rack, for instance). Lie under the bar and grab it with a shoulder-width, overhand grip. Hang at arm's length from the bar with your body in a straight line from your ankles to your shoulders. Pull your chest to the bar as you keep your upper arms perpendicular to your body. Lower yourself and repeat.

V-Up (Instead of Situp)

Works abdominals. This move activates your abdominal muscles from two directions. It requires a rapid contraction of your abdominals and good lower-back and hamstring flexibility.

Lie on your back on the floor with your legs straight. Hold your arms straight above your chest, fingers pointing toward the ceiling. Contract your abdominal muscles and fold your body up by lifting your legs off the floor and stretching your arms toward your toes. Keep your back straight. Pause, then return to the starting position.

How to cheat smart: Perform an "incline reverse crunch." Lie on a slant board with your hips lower than your head, knees slightly bent. Grab the board's handles and pull your hips upward and inward, keeping your knees at the same angle throughout the move. Once you can do three sets of 15 repetitions while holding a 10-pound dumb-bell between your feet, go back to the hanging version.

The benefit: For those who aren't strong enough to do the hanging knee raise with perfect form, the slant-board variation is the best way to cheat without cheating your abs.

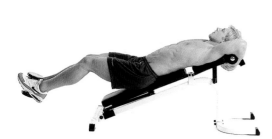

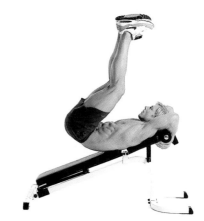

Cardio for the Cut Guy

Because even muscleheads need strong hearts

BY MICHAEL MEJIA, CSCS

You love lifting. You love the plain challenge and the simple rewards—beating your previous best and feeling a great pump afterward.

And maybe you hate cardio. Devoting gym time to cardiovascular exercise feels as if you're burning away hard-earned muscle. But you're not—you're revealing it.

If gaining mass is all you focus on, soon no one will be able to distinguish your traps from your deltoids. For a lean and chiseled physique, you need cardio work. Relax—no distance running involved.

Besides, you know you need aerobic exercise for a healthy heart. And a healthy heart is more efficient at transporting blood and oxygen to working muscles. The stronger your heart, the stronger each of its contractions. That means more oxygenated blood is pumped out with each beat.

What follows is a set of rules to help lifters build healthy hearts. You don't need much cardio work, and most of what you do need should be at high intensity, as befits a man with a lifter's mindset. It'll help you see more muscle definition without wasting time in the gym spinning your wheels.

Rule #1: Change the Cycle

You don't lift the same way all year, so why should the frequency, intensity, and duration of your cardiovascular workouts stay the same? They shouldn't.

When you're trying to add muscle, keep your aerobic work to a minimum—say, once or twice a week for about 15 to 20 minutes. This will limit your energy expenditure and allow your body to concentrate on building muscle.

When you're trying to get lean, increase your cardio training to two to four times a week, to help strip away excess body fat.

At all times, alternate your cardio methods so your workout's not so boring—treadmill running one day, rowing or elliptical training the next, cycling the day after that.

Rule #2: Separate Cardio from Lifting

Serious lifters worry that cardiovascular training will impede their ability to recover from intense strength training. That all depends on when and how you do your cardio.

Keep your cardio days and strength days as removed from each other as possible. That way your cardio won't hinder gains in strength and size. For instance, doing a tough cycling workout after you hammer your legs with squats and lunges isn't a good idea if your goal is to build bigger legs. Save your cardio for the next day, or even the day after that, to rest your legs.

If you must do cardio and weights on the same day, choose a form of aerobic work

PAINkiller

Swallow the Pain
What supplements will help prevent muscle soreness from weight training?

M.F., Kansas City

None have yet been proven effective in preventing muscle soreness. And since anti-inflammatories can limit postexercise muscle building, remember, no pain, no gain. Make that no soreness, no moreness.

that emphasizes body parts your weight lifting didn't focus on that day. So if your cardio choice is rowing, which works your upper body as much as it does your legs, row on a day when your weight session doesn't concentrate on your upper body.

Whichever route you choose, be sure to hit the weights first. You don't want to wipe yourself out before your weight routine—you won't get the most out of your session, and lifting when you're tired can be dangerous.

Rule #3: Don't Make an Impact

Your body has enough to contend with in repairing the damage that lifting inflicts on it. The last thing you need to do is break it down further with high-impact cardio training.

Concentrate on cardio workouts that minimize microtrauma—the small tears to muscle fibers that are part of the process of building new muscle. Running on hard surfaces like asphalt or concrete can be traumatic to muscles and joints. Jumping rope can cause similar problems. Your best bets for low-impact exercise are swimming, cycling, and using an elliptical machine.

Rule #4: Ignore the "Fat-Burning Zone"

It's a myth that you have to work out continuously for 20 minutes before you begin burning fat. The thinking once was that you needed to exercise in a range between 60 and 80 percent of your maximum heart rate. Any lower was too easy; any higher made it too difficult to efficiently use fat for fuel.

Ignore that theory. Your body uses more energy overall when training at high intensities—just look at the physique of a sprinter. Going all out also makes better use of your time. You can finish your cardio in an intense 10- to 15-minute workout.

Stick to interval workouts that feature short bursts of high-intensity movement followed by active recovery periods. (See the sample workouts that follow.) This approach is best for your heart and for fat loss.

Rule #5: Choose the Path of More Resistance

Changing the gears on a bike and altering the gradient on a treadmill, for instance, are great ways to increase intensity. Just be careful to find a level of resistance that won't reduce the amount of work you're able to do when you return to the weight room.

Now that you know the rules, follow these guidelines, depending on your goals.

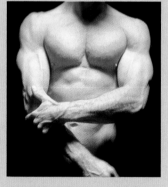

Bulk Cycle (12 weeks)

Do this when you're trying to add muscle.

Frequency: Twice a week

Duration: 10 to 15 minutes (not including warmup and cooldown)

Protocol: Intervals

Intensity: High

Example: Stationary cycling

Warmup: 5 minutes of light pedaling

Work interval: 20 seconds of pedaling as fast as you can

Recovery interval: 40 seconds of light pedaling

Total reps: 10 to 15

Cooldown: 3 to 5 minutes of light pedaling

Lean Cycle (8 weeks)

Do this when you're trying to gain definition.

Frequency: Two to four times a week

Duration: 15 to 20 minutes (not including warmup and cooldown)

Protocol: Intervals

Intensity: High

Example: Rowing

Warmup: 3 to 5 minutes of light rowing

Work interval: 45 seconds of hard rowing

Recovery interval: 90 seconds easy

Total reps: 7 to 9

Cooldown: 3 to 5 minutes of light rowing

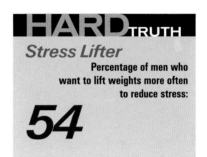

HARD TRUTH

Stress Lifter

Percentage of men who want to lift weights more often to reduce stress:

54

Training Tips

SPLIT THINGS UP

Q **I've had great results lifting 3 days a week. Should I up it to 4?**

T.J., BALTIMORE

A A 4-day split will give you more options to vary your routine. Focus each session on either pulling or pushing movements. For example . . .

Days 1 and 3: Upper-body pushing (bench press, shoulder press, dumbbell fly), lower-body pushing (squat, lunge)

Days 2 and 4: Upper-body pulling (pullup, triceps pulldown, row), lower-body pulling (Romanian deadlift, leg curl)

Don't feel confined to this schedule. Another challenging approach is to do upper push and lower pull on days 1 and 3, then lower push and upper pull on days 2 and 4. When time is short, try a total-body workout twice a week.

GET SET, GROW

Q **I always use heavy weights, but my muscles aren't growing. Isn't heavy lifting supposed to build muscle?**

L.W., ELIZABETH, NEW JERSEY

A Not exactly. To stimulate muscle growth, a set needs to last 40 to 60 seconds, but a typical set of six to eight repetitions lasts only 12 to 20 seconds. Using the same lifting tempo for a set of 15 repetitions with moderate weight would yield more results in terms of muscle growth.

MORE MUSCLE

Are You Iron Deficient?

Many men—beginners especially—might not be lifting as much weight as necessary to build muscle. Researchers at Grand Valley State University in Michigan asked 30 novices to work out with amounts of weight that they thought would help their muscles grow. All of the men chose weight loads below 60 percent of their one-repetition maximums (the heaviest you can lift once). "Lifting less than 60 percent will cause little tissue adaptation," says Stephen Glass, PhD, the lead study author. If you work with only 60 percent of your one-rep max using proper form, he says, you'll probably be able to do 15 to 20 repetitions. To build muscle, you should use weights that won't allow you to do that many.

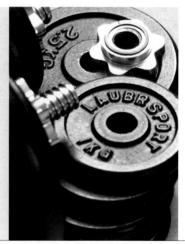

SIZE DOESN'T MATTER

My biceps have grown 2 inches this month, but I still struggle to do a single pullup. Why?

D.K., SAN ANTONIO, TEXAS

You've just learned two key lessons. One: Size doesn't always equal strength. Two: Big biceps don't help much with pullups. If you want to get good at any lift, you have to practice that particular movement. Try using an assisted-pullup machine. Or, recruit your legs for help. Place a step under the bar and push yourself into the up position, then lower yourself as slowly as possible. Shoot for three sets of six repetitions.

ONE AT A TIME

When I do two-handed exercises like the barbell bench press or military press, I lift more with my right hand, and my left hand just picks up the slack. Is this bad?

T.S., ATLANTA

It's not ideal, but it is common. To get your muscles in sync, perform mainly isolateral (one side at a time) movements with dumb-

bells for 3 to 4 weeks. Instead of the barbell bench press, try a dumbbell alternating bench press or a dumbbell single-arm bench press. After this phase, add some of the barbell movements back into your training.

DROP THE GLOVES

Do weight gloves hurt, help, or just look cool?

A.C., NORFOLK, VIRGINIA

None of the above. Gloves mainly protect your hands from developing calluses. Some gloves add texture to increase friction, and others include wrist wraps for support. But look at the serious weight trainers or athletes at your gym—you won't see them in gloves, and they're pretty cool guys.

BALD VERSUS BRAWN

I'm using the baldness drug Propecia, but I've heard that it lowers androgen levels. Will it affect my results at the gym?

E.J., LAS CRUCES, NEW MEXICO

No. This is a common misconception. Propecia (finasteride)

actually blocks the effects of a compound that causes androgen to be converted to alpha-dihydrotestosterone (DHT, aka the cause of balding). Your androgen levels will not go down—the point of the medication is to keep them intact. So your form and follicles should remain strong.

QUICK RECOVERY

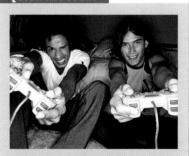

Strong under Pressure

Being muscular can help regulate your blood pressure in stressful situations, according to researchers at the Medical College of Georgia. The researchers measured the BPs of people before, while, and after they played video games. The BPs of men with more muscle mass returned to normal faster than those of the out-of-shape gamers. Researchers say muscle helps excrete sodium, which lowers BP following a spike.

A SPOONFUL OF SUGAR

Q **My creatine supplement has aspartame in it. I've heard that artificial sweeteners can be bad for you. Should I be worried?**

T.J., AIKEN, SOUTH CAROLINA

A Not at all. While there are those who would like to

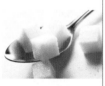

blame aspartame for everything from causing cancer to starting wars, there is conclusive evidence from levelheaded scientific reviews that the artificial sweetener is safe. Plus, you wouldn't want to taste creatine without it. Unless you feel like having your supplement with a scoop of sugar, it's fine to take one that contains aspartame.

IT'S A STRETCH

Q **I have stretch marks from lifting. What can I do?**

S.S., MONTROSE, PENNSYLVANIA

A Unfortunately, very little. No one knows why some people get stretch marks and others—even the friggin' Hulk—don't. Plus, there's no completely effective treatment to prevent them or

make them disappear, says Chris Harmon, MD, a dermatologist in Birmingham, Alabama, who specializes in laser resurfacing. Most stretch marks start off as pink or red streaks that take on the texture of thin cigarette paper. Your best bet is to visit the doctor while they're still red or pink, when a laser treatment might keep them from advancing. (It'll cost you $500 to $1,000, depending on the size of the area treated.) These procedures have a 50 percent success rate (as opposed to nearly useless over-the-counter stretch-mark creams). If it's too late for that, ask your dermatologist about Retin-A creams, which have been partially successful in treating more advanced stretch marks. Meanwhile, look on the bright side—your problem isn't one-tenth the claw marks that the average pregnant woman deals with.

BULK UP

Q **How can a skinny guy with a high metabolism gain weight?**

E.H., ORANGEBURG, NEW YORK

A To achieve Pizza the Huttness, eat 17 large pies with extra cheese per day for a month. But to pack on healthy pounds, eat more and lift weights—the right way to build muscle.

Step 1 Mix one scoop of whey-protein powder into a glass of milk before each workout. Men who take an amino-acid supplement (whey protein is rich in amino acids) before they lift build more muscle than those who fuel up after they exercise. Eat snacks all day, focusing on foods that are high in protein and low in saturated fat, like lean meats, nuts, egg whites, and low-fat dairy products. And have plenty, or your body will eat the muscle you're trying to build. (See the calculator at MensHealth.com/caloriecalc.)

Step 2 Perform exercises that maximize the number of muscles used in each move. This means front squats, seated rows, deadlifts, and incline dumbbell presses. "For skinny guys, isolation exercises are a complete waste of time," says Mike Mejia, CSCS, *Men's Health* contributing editor and coauthor of *Scrawny to Brawny.* Use a heavy weight—something you can lift no more than six times—and stop at five sets.

Bench-Press Boost

When you're stuck bench-pressing the same weight, you've probably worked your pectoralis major so much that your small, stabilizing muscles—your rotator cuffs and the muscles around your neck and shoulder blades—aren't working well enough.

The fix: After your bench-press routine, do up to three sets of 8 to 12 reps of the moves below, resting 60 seconds between sets. Keep your quads and glutes tight; pull your navel toward your spine. You should see up to a 15 percent gain in chest strength in 4 weeks. If you're new to weight lifting, do only the first exercise after you bench-press; do the first two if you have some experience; and do all three if you're more advanced.

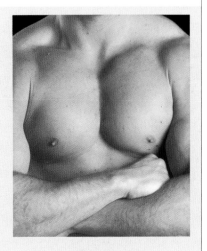

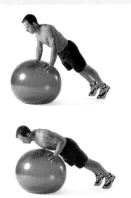

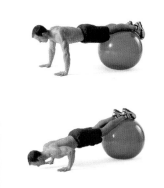

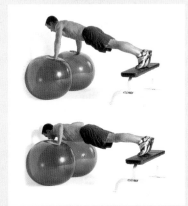

Swiss-Ball Incline Pushup
With your toes on the floor, assume the standard pushup position, but place your hands on a Swiss ball directly under your shoulders. Bend your arms until your chest touches the ball. Pause, then push yourself back up to the starting position.

Swiss-Ball Decline Pushup
This time, position yourself so your shins are resting on a Swiss ball and your hands are on the floor. Tuck your chin and, leading with your chest, lower your body until your arms form 90-degree angles.

Double Swiss-Ball Pushup
Set two Swiss balls against a wall a few feet in front of a bench. Place a hand on the center of each ball, making sure the balls are touching, and rest your feet on the bench. Lower your body as far as you can with control. Pause, then push yourself back up to the starting position.

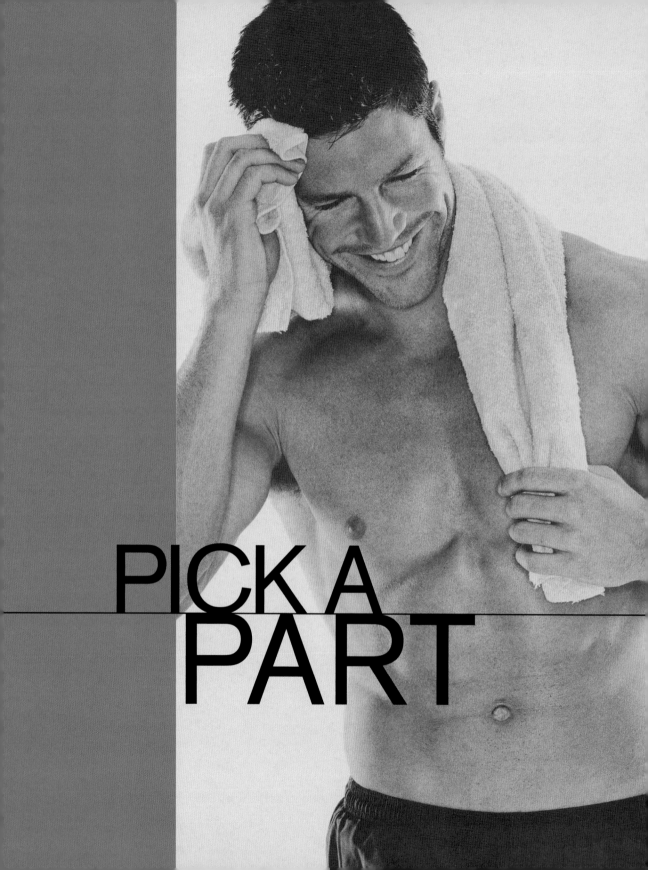

PICK A PART

Everyone's looking to get something different from his workout, be it a muscular physique, stress relief, or a date with the towel girl at the gym. But most guys are looking to look more ripped. And by ripped, 57 percent of guys say they mean they want a six-pack. A third equate looking ripped with boasting big arms. And another 27 percent say it means having chiseled pecs.

No matter which muscles you associate with being ripped, you'll find a workout here to bulk them up. From abs and arms to shoulders and legs, we've got you covered. Just pick a part and start reading, and you're one step closer to getting the look you're after.

BY MYATT MURPHY

Ab Salute

Sit up and take notice

If you've been diligently working your midsection but remain a few cans shy of a six-pack, there may be a simple explanation. You need the right diet and exercise program (weights and cardiovascular) to burn off fat before you can develop a cover-model stomach. But even before you whittle down that fatty layer, you should condition your abdominal muscles with a few good moves that isolate your midsection. It's wise to save your abdominal routine for the end of your workout, since your ab muscles help stabilize your waist during many exercises for other muscle groups.

The Payoff

Extra power. Exercising your ab muscles using moves that involve twisting at the waist can build the kind of rotational strength your midsection needs for delivering extra power when you throw, punch, or swing.

Perfect posture. Tight lower-back muscles from excessive running pull your spine out of its natural alignment. Strengthening your abdominal wall can correct this muscular imbalance, improving your body's posture to allow it to function more efficiently.

Less pain. The weaker your abdominal muscles, the more your lower back has to compensate to support your body. Keeping the abs strong can balance the workload and protect your back from strains and pulls.

Better protection. Most abdominal exercises work the transverse abdominis, a thin band of muscle that supports and protects your internal organs.

The Main Move

The most popular abdominal exercise—the crunch—remains one of the best ways to sculpt an amazing midsection.

THE CRUNCH

Lie on your back with your knees bent and your feet flat on the floor, about hip-width apart. Place your hands so that they lightly touch your head behind your ears. As you begin to exhale, slowly curl your head and torso toward your knees until your shoulder blades are off the floor. Imagine that you're drawing your ribs to your hips, as if your midsection were an accordion. Pause, then return to the starting position, inhaling as you go.

Perfect Form

Head: Keep your head in alignment with your spine. (Turning it to either side tightens the neck muscles and places them at risk of strain.) Your eyes should always look up and slightly forward. If you're looking at your knees as you curl, you're probably tilting your head too far forward.

Hands: Don't lace your hands behind your head—you'll be tempted to tug on your neck. Place your fingers lightly behind your ears, or cross your hands on your chest.

Mouth: Breathe normally through your mouth. Exhaling forcefully as you crunch can cause you to lose energy instead of conserving it. Inhale as you lower yourself and exhale as you rise.

Shoulders: Most people roll their shoulders up and forward, which places strain on the upper back and neck while making the crunch easier and less effective. Instead, concentrate on folding your upper body forward, keeping your shoulders and upper back straight (not rounded) as you crunch.

Abs: Suck in your stomach muscles. Keeping them in a constant state of contraction throughout the exercise strengthens your transverse abdominis, the thin band of muscle that runs across your midsection. A strong transverse abdominis can improve your posture to create the effect of flatter abs.

Back: Don't lift yourself up more than 45 degrees. Beyond this point, you're using more of your back and hip flexors instead of your abs to perform the work.

Lower back: Your tailbone and lower back should stay in contact with the floor throughout the exercise. If you feel your lower back leaving the ground, you've raised yourself farther than is necessary to isolate your abdominal muscles.

Feet: Space your feet about hip-width apart and plant them firmly on the floor. Don't hook them under anything. Anchoring your feet transfers more of the stress from your abdominals to your hip flexors—the muscles that attach the front of your torso to your legs.

Mix and Max

Raise your feet for more results. The traditional crunch relies mostly on the upper part of your rectus abdominis—the muscle group that makes up your six-pack—and places less emphasis on the lower rectus. To involve the lower portion more, keep your knees bent, but suspend your feet an inch off the floor instead of planting them flat.

Touch your chest before you rest. Where you place your hands can change the degree of difficulty of a crunch. If you can't complete the last repetition of a set, try moving your hands from behind your ears to across your chest. This displaces a portion of your weight and may allow you to do one or two more crunches and work the muscles a little longer.

Increase the resistance. The fitter you are, the less body weight you probably have to use as resistance, making ab exercises easier and less effective. Using weight plates, medicine balls, or pulleys can help you exhaust your abdominal muscles.

The Workout

We talk about six-packs, but the real number is four—your abdominal muscles are divided into four distinct groups. These six exercises hit them all, while giving you enough variety to keep things interesting. After the crunch, pick one exercise from each section: A (upper and lower rectus ab-

The Right Workout for You
Sculpt amazing abs with our easy-to-use checklist

YOUR LEVEL	WORK YOUR ABS	SETS OF EACH EXERCISE	REPETITIONS PER SET	SPEED OF EACH REP	REST BETWEEN SETS
Beginner	Three times a week	2–3	10–15	3–4 seconds up, 3–4 seconds down	30–60 seconds
Intermediate	Twice a week	2–4	10–15	3–4 seconds up, 3–4 seconds down	60–90 seconds
Advanced	Twice a week	3–5	10–15	3–4 seconds up, 3–4 seconds down	90–240 seconds

dominis, or a portion of the rectus abdominis and the obliques) and B (upper and lower rectus abdominis, plus obliques). Remember to pull your stomach in as you exercise and you'll incorporate the transverse abdominis. To really isolate the transverse abdominis, add exercise C. Whichever moves you choose, you'll hit your abs from several angles to build a strong, flat midsection that works hard and looks even harder.

WEIGHTED CRUNCH (A)
Works entire rectus abdominis

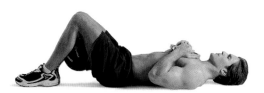

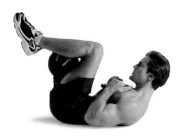

Lie flat on your back with your knees bent and your feet flat on the floor. Place a light medicine ball between your knees and squeeze it so it stays in place throughout the exercise. Hold a light weight plate (5 to 8 pounds to start) in your hands. Slowly draw your knees up toward your chest while simultaneously curling your head and shoulders off the ground. Pause, then slowly lower your legs and upper body back to the floor, or just above the floor to keep constant tension on your rectus abdominis.

Get more: Instead of a weight plate, hold a medicine ball at your chest, keeping your elbows out to your sides. Have your workout partner stand in front of you. As you curl up, throw the ball to your partner. Ask him to lightly toss the ball back at your chest so you can catch it, pull it back to your body, and then curl back down.

CABLE PULLDOWN (A)
Works upper rectus abdominis, obliques

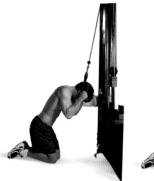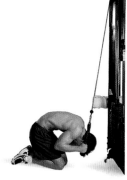

Kneel in front of a high-pulley cable and grab a rope attachment with both hands. Position your hands either by your ears (palms facing in) or just below your chin (palms touching the top of your chest). Keeping your hands locked in place, slowly curl yourself down and forward, starting by drawing your chin toward your chest, then letting your shoulders and back follow. Curl down as far as you comfortably can, then slowly reverse the motion. After each repetition done in this way, curl yourself down while twisting either to the left or to the right. Alternate sides on each repetition to work your obliques.

Get more: Stand with your right shoulder facing the machine. Reach your left arm across your face and grab the handle, then place your right hand on top of your left hand. Rotate your torso to your left as you draw your arms across and down. Once your hands are above your left thigh, slowly return to the starting position. Switch sides and repeat.

PULSE TWIST (A)

Works lower rectus abdominis, obliques

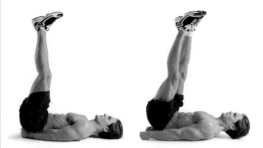

Lie on your back and tuck your hands under your pelvis, along the sides of your tailbone. Keeping your legs straight and feet together, raise them so the soles of your feet point toward the ceiling and your buttocks lift a few inches off the floor. At the top of the move, twist your hips to the right so that your feet point to the left. Lower your legs back to the starting position and repeat the move, this time twisting your hips to the left.

Get more: Instead of twisting your hips at the top of the move, lower your butt to the floor, then slowly roll both legs to one side. Go as far as you comfortably can without losing your balance. Rotate your legs back up until they're above your hips and repeat the exercise, this time lowering your legs to the other side.

TWISTING LEGS-UP CRUNCH (B)

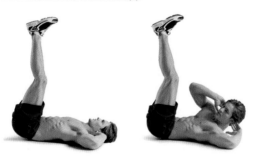

Lie on your back and raise your legs so that the soles of your feet point toward the ceiling. Place

your hands lightly behind your ears, elbows pointing out. Keeping your legs upright, slowly curl up and to the left. Lower yourself and repeat to the right. Alternate from left to right throughout the set.

Get more: Start the move with your legs straight and suspended at a 45-degree angle to the floor. As you curl your upper body off the floor, simultaneously raise your legs until your feet point toward the ceiling. As you bring your head and shoulders back down to the floor, lower your legs back to a 45-degree angle.

TWISTING CRUNCH (B)

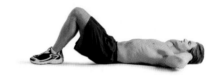

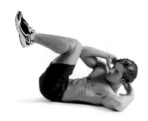

Lie on your back with your legs bent at 90 degrees and your feet on the floor. Touch your hands lightly to the sides of your head. Slowly lift your shoulders off the ground and twist your body to the left so your right elbow points between your knees. At the same time, draw your knees up and in to meet the elbow. Lower yourself back down and repeat the move, this time twisting to the right so that your left elbow points between your knees.

Get more: Attach a bar to the end of a low-pulley cable and lie with your feet pointing toward it. Wrap your feet underneath the bar and raise your legs till they point straight up. The bar should rest along your insteps, with the cable between your feet. Now do twisting crunches, feeling the constant tension on the lower portion of your abs.

SWISS-BALL STABILITY POSE (C)

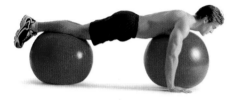

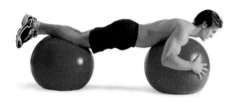

Grab two Swiss balls and lie facedown across them. Your body should be straight, with just your chest lying on the first ball and your knees and shins resting on the other. With your feet spaced about 12 to 18 inches apart, place your hands on the floor for balance and hold this position for 60 seconds.

Get more: As the stability pose becomes easy, place your hands on the sides of the ball. For a greater challenge, try reaching your arms out to the sides or straightening them in front of your head. Moving your feet in closer together so they touch also increases the difficulty.

Challenging Changeups

Long-Arm Crunch
Lie with your arms straightened behind your head, hands clasped together. As you curl up, keep your arms in line with your upper body—your upper arms should touch your ears at all times. Having part of the weight of your arms farther away from your body adds resistance to the move when you don't have any plates or balls handy.

Medicine-Ball Crunch
Lie with your feet flat on the floor, knees bent at a 90-degree angle. Instead of placing your hands alongside your head, hold a medicine ball against your chest with both hands. This adds resistance more comfortably than holding a weight plate.

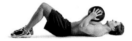 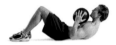

Swiss-Ball Crunch
Sit on top of a Swiss ball with your legs in front of you, feet flat on the floor. Slowly lean back and roll yourself down the ball until just your shoulder blades and back touch. Then perform crunches. This forces your muscles to contract before you begin the move.

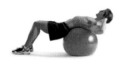

Low-Pulley Cable Crunch
Lie on your back in front of a low-pulley station and attach a rope to the cable. Lie back in the standard crunch position, your head toward the pulley, then reach back and grab one end of the rope in each hand. Tuck your fists by your chest and curl. This variation is ideal for lighter guys who need to add the right amount of resistance to thoroughly work their abs.

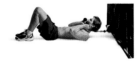 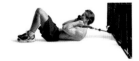

Meet Your Muscles

Your abdominals are composed of four muscle groups: the rectus abdominis (1), the external (2) and internal obliques (3), and the transverse abdominis (4). Together, these four muscle groups support the torso and assist it in various movements—bending the body to either side, twisting right and left, and lowering and raising the upper body.

The rectus abdominis, which is responsible for pulling your torso toward your hips, attaches at your sternum and your fifth through seventh ribs, and connects to your pubic bone. The external obliques run diagonally down from the lower ribs and connect to the pelvis and the pubic bone.

The internal obliques, which lie underneath the external obliques and run diagonally to them, start on the iliac crest and connect to your lower three ribs. The internal and external obliques are responsible for torso rotation and lateral flexion (bending to the side).

Finally, the transverse abdominis muscle, which runs underneath your obliques, stretches from your lower ribs to your pubic bone. Its main job is to pull your abdominal wall inward, protecting your internal organs and helping you expel air.

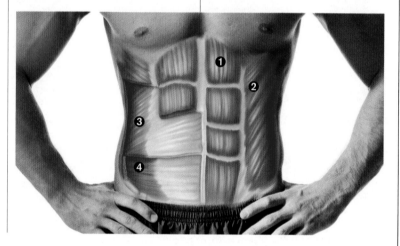

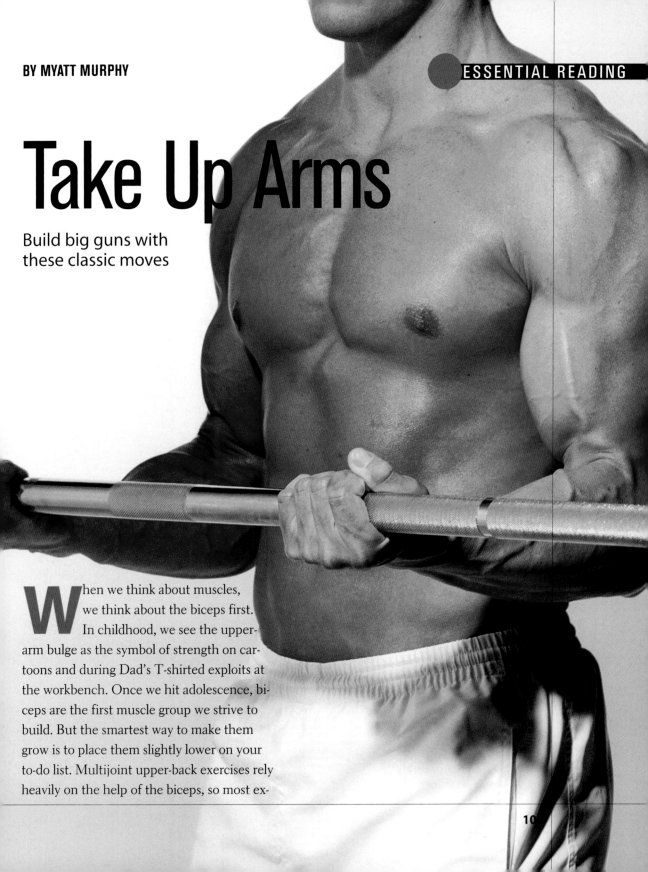

BY MYATT MURPHY

Take Up Arms

Build big guns with
these classic moves

When we think about muscles, we think about the biceps first. In childhood, we see the upper-arm bulge as the symbol of strength on cartoons and during Dad's T-shirted exploits at the workbench. Once we hit adolescence, biceps are the first muscle group we strive to build. But the smartest way to make them grow is to place them slightly lower on your to-do list. Multijoint upper-back exercises rely heavily on the help of the biceps, so most experts recommend working your back and biceps in the same workout. If you prefer exercising them on separate days, allow at least 48 hours of rest after each workout, or your biceps won't have enough time to recover and grow.

The Payoff

Attention getter. The biceps are one of the few muscle groups you can expose almost anywhere, anytime. Sculpted arms make others inclined to assume the rest of you is chiseled as well.

A wider back. Back exercises require a lot of help from your biceps. So the stronger your biceps are, the more weight you'll be able to use when training your back.

A stronger grip. Nearly all of the exercises that work your biceps also strengthen the tendons and muscles throughout your wrists and hands, leaving you with a firmer, more powerful handshake.

A perfect stride. Pumping your arms as you run is crucial to maintaining an even rhythm. Strong biceps can improve your pace by giving you more control of your arm swing.

Dynamic sex. To pull off certain sexual positions that require and show off your strength (we're thinking wheelbarrow or any standing variation), well-built biceps will support her legs for as long as it takes.

The Main Move

Nothing adds size and shape to the biceps like the barbell curl, a move that lets you lift more weight than any other biceps exercise.

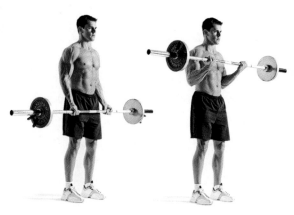

BARBELL CURL

Grab a barbell with an underhand grip (palms up), your hands shoulder-width apart. Your arms should hang straight so the bar is directly in front of your thighs. Keeping your back straight and abdominals drawn in, curl the bar up in a semicircular motion until your forearms touch your biceps. Pause, then slowly lower the bar to the starting position.

Perfect Form

Head: Always keep your head in line with your upper back. Turning your head to the side (to look at your biceps) or tilting it down (to see the bar) can strain neck muscles that are already contracted during the exercise. If you need to check your form, stand in front of a mirror.

Shoulders: At the top of the curl, your fists should end up directly in front of your shoulders. If your fists stop either above or below them, you're not keeping your upper arms against your body.

Upper arms: Keep them tucked tightly into your body throughout the move. Moving them forward as you curl indicates that you're probably arching your back. Pushing them out to the sides moves your wrists out of alignment with your forearms, which can place stress on the wrist tendons.

Biceps: At the top of the move, flex your biceps for 1 to 2 seconds before lowering the weight.

Elbows: Your elbows should stay close to your body and point at the floor. If they shift forward or out to the sides, you're compromising your posture to lift the weight by using other muscles.

Forearms: Your forearms should be the only parts of your body that move during the exercise. Curl the bar high enough to bring the upper ends of your forearms to your biceps.

Wrists: Keep your wrists in line with your forearms throughout the exercise. Allowing the weight to pull your wrists downward as you curl places stress on the tendons in your wrists.

Hands: Grab the bar with an underhand grip with your hands about shoulder-width apart. As you curl, maintain a firm grip, but don't overdo it—gripping the bar too tightly can cause your hands to tire before your biceps are finished working.

Back: Your spine should stay in line throughout the move. Arching backward or forward places stress on your lower back.

Legs: As you lower the bar, bring it down just in front of your thighs, but never rest the bar against your legs. Resting the bar reduces the tension on your biceps that you want to maintain throughout the move.

Knees: Keep them unlocked at all times, but never bent. If you feel yourself bending your knees at any point during the exercise, you could be cheating by creating upward momentum.

Feet: Keep your feet shoulder-width apart and flat on the floor. Rising up on your toes or leaning back on your heels compromises your stability and means you're trying to use momentum to cheat the weight up.

Mix and Max

Change your spacing. Move your hands a few inches closer together to stress more of the outer part of your biceps. Move them farther apart to place more emphasis on the inner part.

Wrap it up. Place a towel around the bar to force your hands, wrists, and forearms to work harder to keep a tight grip, so you're strengthening them as you curl.

Get on your knees. Reduce the weight you typically use by 20 percent and try the

PEAK
performance

Kick Back for Big Biceps

Training your triceps can help your biceps grow stronger. Australian researchers reviewed 13 studies that examined how training one muscle affects its contralateral, or opposite, muscle. They found that after at least 2 weeks of training a particular muscle, men and women increased strength in the opposite muscle by 8 percent. Study authors say the mechanism behind this effect is unclear. But it's worth a shot: Lay off the biceps curls for a couple of weeks and try some triceps kickbacks, dips, or pulldowns.

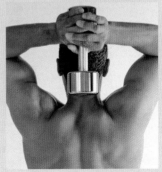

exercise from a kneeling position. This makes it more difficult to use momentum to cheat the weight up, and it focuses more of the effort on your biceps and less on your lower back.

The Workout

Building impressive biceps is easier than you think. Unlike muscle groups that require many exercises to work them from several angles, the biceps are somewhat limited in their mobility. The curl is the best exercise, but that doesn't mean you can't be creative. Designing a mix of moves that strengthen your biceps as well as your brachialis and forearm muscles can keep your workouts interesting and your arms growing. After doing the barbell curl, pick one exercise from section A (biceps) and one from B (biceps/brachialis/forearms). Then build your program according to the chart below. Whatever mix you pick, this plan will give you the guns you've been looking for.

PREACHER CURL (A)

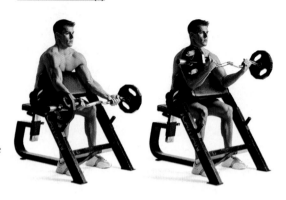

Sit at a preacher-curl station and grab a pair of light dumbbells or an EZ-curl bar with an underhand grip. Rest your upper arms on the slanted pad in front of you. Keeping your back straight, slowly curl the bar up until your forearms are just short of perpendicular to the floor. Then lower the weight back down.

Get more: Move the preacher station in front of a low-cable pulley and try doing cable curls using the bench. The resistance will come from the angle rather than from the downward force of gravity, so you'll work the muscle fibers differently.

The Right Workout for You

Build a set of perfect biceps with our easy checklist

YOUR LEVEL	WORK YOUR BICEPS	SETS OF EACH EXERCISE	REPETITIONS PER SET	SPEED OF EACH REP	REST BETWEEN SETS
Beginner	Three times a week	1–3	10–15	3–4 seconds up, 3–4 seconds down	30–60 seconds
Intermediate	Twice a week	2–4	8–12	2–3 seconds up, 2–3 seconds down	60–120 seconds
Advanced	Twice a week	3–5	6–8	2 seconds up, 2 seconds down	90–40 seconds

CONCENTRATION CURL (A)

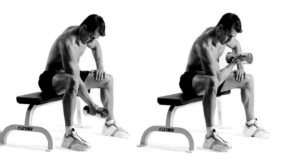

Sit on the edge of a bench with a dumbbell in your right hand, your legs spread out to the sides. Rest the back of your right arm against the inside of your right thigh. Hold the weight with an underhand grip and let it hang straight down. Rest your left hand on your left thigh. Curl the weight up toward your right shoulder. Pause, then lower the weight to the starting position.

Get more: Before you curl, try rotating your hand inward until the knuckle of your thumb points toward the opposite leg. Curling the weight up this way lets you incorporate the brachialis muscle, underneath your biceps, to add extra size to your arms.

DUMBBELL CURL (A)

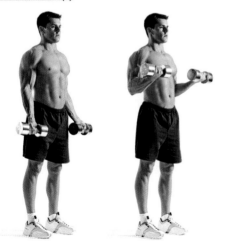

Stand holding a dumbbell in each hand with an underhand grip, arms at your sides. Keeping your upper arms against your sides, slowly curl the weights up until your forearms touch your biceps. Hold the contraction and squeeze your biceps for a second, then slowly lower the weights.

Get more: At the start, turn your palms 180 degrees inward so they face behind you. As you lift, twist your wrists inward so your palms face your shoulders at the top of the move. This forces your wrists, forearms, biceps, and brachialis to assist.

DUMBBELL HAMMER CURL (B)

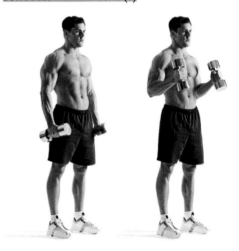

Stand with a dumbbell in each hand, your arms straight down at your sides and your palms facing each other. With your back straight, slowly curl the dumbbells toward your shoulders, keeping your wrists from turning as you go. Your thumbs should point toward your shoulders at the top of the move. Slowly lower the weights to the starting position.

Get more: Try holding the weights farther forward, with the tops of the dumbbells flat against your thumb and forefinger. This gives your forearms a break so they don't give out before your biceps.

REVERSE BARBELL CURL (B)

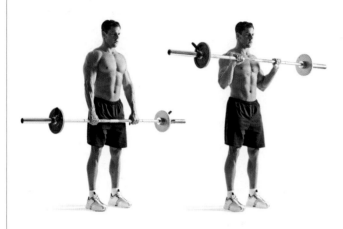

Stand holding a barbell with a shoulder-width, overhand grip, your arms hanging straight down so the bar rests in front of your thighs. Keeping your back straight and elbows tucked into your sides, slowly curl the bar up until your forearms touch your biceps. Pause, then slowly lower the bar to the starting position.

Get more: Once you become proficient, try this using a pair of dumbbells. You'll find it takes more effort to maintain proper form.

Meet Your Muscles

The front of your upper arm owes its bulge to two muscle groups—the biceps brachii and the brachialis.

The biceps brachii muscle (1) covers the front part of your upper arm and has two sections, or heads (hence the prefix "bi," meaning "two"). The long head—also called the outer head—attaches by way of the biceps tendon to the scapula, or shoulder blade, at a point (the glenoid cavity) deep inside the shoulder capsule. The short head stems from a bony hook (the coracoid) near the top of the scapula. The two muscles join below the shoulder, and their combined end attaches to the radius, one

of two major bones of the forearm.

The brachialis (2) is sandwiched between the humerus (the bone in your upper arm) and the biceps. Developing this

unseen sinew gives it no place to go but up, pushing the biceps higher. Together, the biceps and brachialis are responsible for flexing your arm and turning your palm and forearm up.

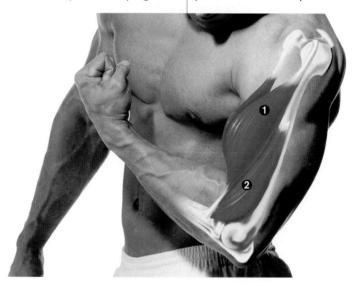

WRIST EXTENSION (B)

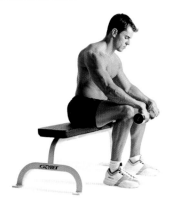

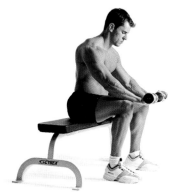

Sit on a bench with your knees bent, feet shoulder-width apart. Grab a very light dumbbell in each hand and place your forearms on your thighs, palms down, so your wrists are hanging over your knees. (You may have to lean forward slightly to get your forearms flat against your legs.) Bending at the wrists, lower the dumbbells as far as possible while keeping a tight grip. Now raise the weights as high as you can, keeping your forearms pressed against your thighs throughout the move. Return to the starting position.

Get more: Turn your hands over so that your palms face up. This position works the bottom of your forearms (the wrist flexors), whereas raising the weights with your palms down develops the top portion (the wrist extensors).

Challenging Changeups

Incline Dumbbell Curl

Lie faceup on an incline bench and hold a pair of dumbbells in each hand with an underhand grip, allowing your arms to hang straight down. Keeping your upper arms stationary, slowly curl the weights up until they reach the outside of your chest. Starting with your arms behind your body this way works your muscles differently.

EZ-Curl-Bar Curl

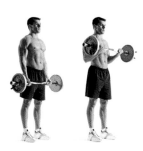

The series of bends on an EZ-curl bar is designed to relieve stress on your wrists. The bar lets you use a wider or narrower grip without placing added stress on your tendons, and its shorter length makes it easier to balance the weight as you curl.

Behind-the-Back One-Arm Cable Curl

Stand with your back to the weight stack of a cable station and grab the bottom stirrup handle with one hand. Take a few steps away from the stack so there is resistance and your arm is roughly 45 degrees from horizontal. Slowly curl the handle forward and up until your hand reaches the side of your chest. Then lower your arm to the starting position. This stretches your biceps beyond its usual range of motion.

Two-Handed Cable Curl

Attach a short bar to a low-cable pulley and stand 1 to 2 feet from the weight stack. Because you use a closer grip and the resistance comes from an angle, you work the muscle fibers of the biceps differently.

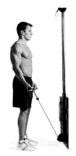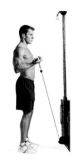

Tri This On for Size

When it comes to larger upper arms, the secret isn't working the muscles in front; it's targeting the larger, stronger triceps behind. The triceps are a secondary muscle group that assists in every exercise you perform for your chest and shoulders. If you train your triceps before your shoulders and chest, the triceps will be the first muscles to quit when you begin your chest or shoulder routine, preventing the latter muscles from being challenged enough to grow. The smartest order: chest first, shoulders second, triceps last.

The Payoff

Bigger arms. Most men target their biceps when trying to build larger arms, but it's the triceps that make up close to 60 percent of the upper arm. Focusing on them can pack on size fast.

More power. The responsibility for throwing, punching, swinging, or pushing off starts with your chest and ends with your triceps. Strong triceps give you an extra burst of strength whenever you straighten your arms—power that makes all the difference in edging out your competition.

Less risk. The triceps protect your elbow joints by acting as shock absorbers, lessening stress whenever your elbows are forced to flex suddenly, such as in breaking your fall in football or bracing yourself on a bumpy trail when mountain biking.

A better body. Most chest and shoulder exercises rely heavily on the triceps as a secondary muscle to help move weight. If you strengthen them, they won't give up before they should, so you'll achieve bigger and better gains with your chest and shoulder routines.

The Main Move

The triceps pushdown is one of the most efficient isolation exercises you can use for improving the size and strength of your triceps muscles.

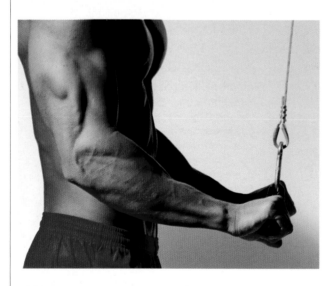

TRICEPS PUSHDOWN

Stand in front of a high-pulley cable station and grab a straight bar with an overhand grip, your hands shoulder-width apart. Keeping your back straight, tuck your upper arms into your sides and position your forearms almost parallel to the floor (hands a bit higher than elbows). Your elbows should be pointing straight behind you. Slowly push the bar down until your arms are straight and the bar reaches your thighs. Pause, then slowly allow the bar to rise until your forearms are again just past parallel to the floor.

Meet Your Muscles

Your triceps are made up of three separate muscles—the lateral head, the medial head, and the long head.

The lateral head (1) attaches to the back of the humerus (your upper-arm bone) and forms the outer side of your triceps. It makes up most of the horseshoe shape of the muscle. The medial head (2) is located along the middle of the back of your upper arm and also attaches to the humerus. The long head (3) is located along the inside of your arm and attaches to the scapula (shoulder blade).

All three heads connect to a tendon attached to the ulna (one of the two bones of the forearm). Together, the three heads are responsible for extending the elbow (straightening your arm). The long head also helps stabilize the underside of your shoulder joint and assists your upper-back muscles in arm adduction (bringing your arm down and in toward your body).

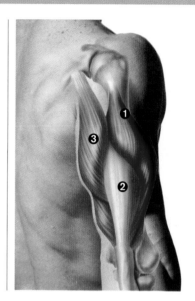

Perfect Form

Head: Keep your head in line with your back throughout the move. Looking down stresses your neck and trapezius muscles and makes it easier to hunch forward to use your shoulder muscles more than your triceps.

Eyes: Fix your gaze straight ahead and resist the urge to look down at the bar as you push. Tilting your chin downward can stress the muscles in your neck and upper back.

Upper arms: Keep them tucked into your sides throughout the move. Flaring them out places more stress on your elbows; pulling them behind you makes it easier to press the weight down using muscles other than your triceps.

Elbows: Your elbows should remain pinned at your sides throughout the move.

Raising them or letting them drift behind you as you push the bar down brings more of your shoulder muscles into the exercise.

Forearms: Your forearms should be just above parallel to the floor at the start of the move. As you push the bar down, keep them straight so they're in line with your shoulders—if they angle out, you could strain your wrists or compromise your posture to use more of your shoulder muscles.

Hands: Hold the bar with your hands shoulder-width apart, palms facing down. Try to position the bar so that it rests mainly against the palms of your hands.

Wrists: Don't let your wrists bend back. Keeping them in line with your forearms places the effort more directly on your triceps and spares the tendons in your wrists.

Lower back: Maintain a straight back throughout the lift. Leaning or hunching forward changes the angle to involve more of the lower-chest and shoulder muscles.

Legs: Your legs should remain slightly bent throughout the exercise.

Feet: Both feet should be pressed flat on the floor at all times. Rising up on your toes probably means you're leaning forward to enlist the help of your shoulder muscles.

Mix and Max

Vary your grip. Moving your hands closer together places more effort on the lateral head of your triceps. Spacing them more than shoulder-width apart works the long and medial heads.

Change tools. If using a straight bar feels uncomfortable for your wrists, try attaching a V-shaped bar to the pulley instead. The move will feel as if you're pushing and pulling at the same time, but by angling your hands toward each other, the V bar will make the motion less stressful for your wrists.

Adjust your approach. A weight stack is ideal for "drop sets" of the triceps pushdown to fatigue your muscles for maximum gains. After your last regular set, lower the weight by one or two plates and perform another set of as many repetitions as you can do. Work your way up the stack until there's one plate left.

The Workout

To develop perfect triceps, it's critical to work them at an assortment of angles. Every triceps exercise calls on all of the three heads that make up the muscle, but some work one head more than the others. In addition to the triceps pushdown, pick one or two exercises from the six that follow, then build your program using the table below. By frequently changing your workout using these six moves, in the long run you'll thoroughly involve all three

The Right Workout for You

Build a set of perfect triceps with our easy-to-use chart

YOUR LEVEL	WORK YOUR TRICEPS	SETS OF EACH EXERCISE	REPETITIONS PER SET	SPEED OF EACH REP	REST BETWEEN SETS
Beginner	Three times a week	1–3	10–15	3–4 seconds up, 3–4 seconds down	30–60 seconds
Intermediate	Twice a week	2–4	8–12	2–3 seconds up, 2–3 seconds down	60–120 seconds
Advanced	Twice a week	3–5	6–8	2 seconds up, 2 seconds down	90–240 seconds

heads of the triceps. The result will be bigger, stronger arms that work well—and look great.

BENCH DIP

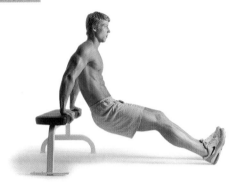

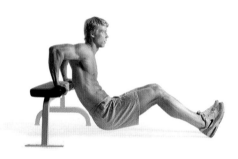

Place your hands on the edge of a bench, fingers pointing toward your lower back. Keeping your hands in place, slowly step forward until your legs are extended in front of you, knees slightly bent. Your arms should be straight, elbows unlocked, supporting your weight. Slowly bend your arms to lower yourself as far as you can and bring your butt as close to the floor as possible. Press yourself back up to the starting position.

Get more: Try resting your heels on another bench. Once that becomes easy, have a spotter place a weight plate across the tops of your thighs with your feet on the floor. Then try the move with a plate across your thighs and your heels on a bench.

Challenging Changeups

Rope Pulldown

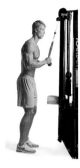
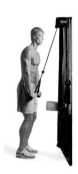

Use a rope attachment instead of a bar. Grab each end of the rope so your palms face each other. Pull the rope down until your arms are straight, turning your wrists inward at the bottom. This variation works all three heads of the triceps more evenly.

Reverse-Grip Triceps Pulldown

Inverting your grip so your palms are up changes the move from a pushing exercise to a pulling one. This places extra stress on the lateral head of the triceps (the most difficult head to develop). Because this muscle lies along the outer edge of the upper arm, hitting it can make your arms look larger from the front and back.

Single-Arm Pulldown/Pushdown

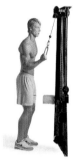
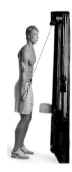

This lets you use a hand to spot yourself. Attach a single handle to a high pulley and grab it with one hand, with your palm facing either up (to pull the weight down) or down (to press the weight down).

Incline Triceps Pushdown

To keep from leaning forward, place an incline bench close to a high-pulley cable, facing away from the machine. Lie flat, grab the bar overhead with an overhand grip, and pull your elbows down until your upper arms are along the sides of your body. Push the bar down until your arms are nearly straight, then slowly return the bar to your chest.

CLOSE-GRIP BENCH PRESS

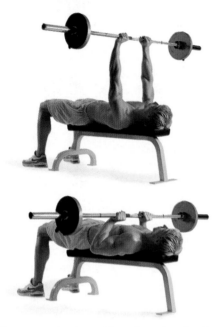

Lie on your back on a bench and grab a barbell with an overhand grip, your hands less than shoulder-width apart and arms extended. Slowly lower the bar to your chest. Pause, then press the weight back overhead, but keep your elbows unlocked.

Get more: Switch the barbell with a pair of dumbbells. Holding your arms straight above your chest, touch the ends of the weights together. Try to keep the ends touching throughout the exercise.

KNEELING CABLE EXTENSION

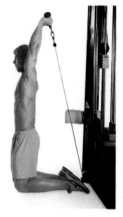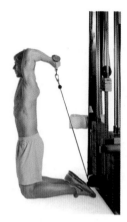

Attach a V bar to a low-pulley cable and kneel with your back to the stack. Turn around to grab both handles, then face forward and straighten your arms overhead. (The bottom of the V should be pointing down.) Keeping your upper arms stationary, slowly bend your elbows and lower your hands behind your neck. Reverse the motion, straightening your arms and locking your elbows at the top to contract the triceps.

Get more: Lie on an incline bench facing away from the low pulley. Grab the rope and raise your arms straight up. Keeping your upper arms perpendicular to the floor, bend your elbows and lower your hands to the sides of your head. Return to the starting position.

LYING DUMBBELL EXTENSION

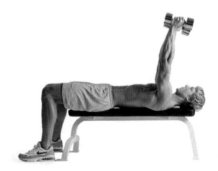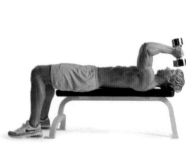

Hold a set of light dumbbells overhead with your arms straight and your palms facing each other. Keeping your upper arms stationary, slowly lower the weights toward your shoulders until they reach the sides of your head. Pause, then slowly press the weights back up, keeping your elbows unlocked.

Get more: Hold one dumbbell with your palm facing your body. Place your other hand on your raised arm's triceps to support it. Bending at the elbow, slowly lower the weight until it touches the front of your opposite shoulder, then raise it back up.

SINGLE-ARM EXTENSION

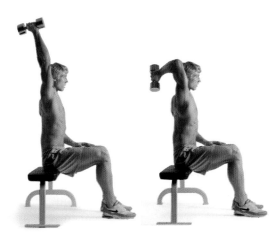

Sit on a bench with a light dumbbell in your right hand. Raise the weight over your head, with your palm facing in. Press your right upper arm against the side of your head and use your left hand to support your right elbow, or place it on your thigh. Slowly lower the weight behind your head as far as you can. Pause, then raise the weight to the starting position. Finish one set, then switch hands.

Get more: At the start of the exercise, rotate your hand so that your palm faces forward. Lower the weight in front of your body instead of behind it, so the end of the dumbbell lightly touches the top of your chest. Then return to the starting position.

TWISTING KICKBACK

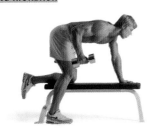

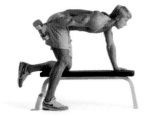

With your left hand and knee resting on a bench, hold a light dumbbell in your right hand. Let your right arm hang down toward the floor, palm facing the bench. Draw the weight close to your body by bringing up your upper arm parallel to the floor and bending your elbow 90 degrees. Keeping your upper arm stationary, slowly straighten the arm. As you go, turn your wrist so that your palm ends up facing the ceiling. Pause and reverse.

Get more: Place the bench lengthwise in front of a low-pulley cable station. With your head toward the pulley, grab one end of the rope with your right hand and perform the exercise as described above. This keeps your triceps contracted throughout the move.

BY MYATT MURPHY

Shoulder Heavier Loads

Be head and shoulders above other guys with these deltoid-delivering exercises

Having great arms, a muscular back, and a powerful chest may seem ideal, but without a strong set of shoulders, you can't build any of them to their full potential—or take advantage of their strength after all your hard work. Your shoulders are secondary muscle groups that assist in most exercises for your chest, back, biceps, and triceps. Since your shoulders are used more during chest exercises, training the chest and shoulders on the same day is the most practical approach. The smartest order: chest first, shoulders second, arms last.

The Payoff

Perfect posture. Having the posterior deltoids significantly weaker than the anterior (front) ones can pull your shoulders forward and down. Keeping the anterior, middle, and posterior fibers strong helps to stabilize your shoulder girdle and keep your shoulders in alignment.

More power. Because of their connection to other muscles, stronger shoulders give you extra strength in almost every exercise you use to work your pectorals, back, biceps, and triceps.

A thinner waist. Broad shoulders create the illusion that you have a smaller waist than you actually do.

Injury prevention. The posterior deltoids are responsible for decelerating your arms every time you throw or swing. Not being able to effectively slow down your arms places more stress on your elbow joints.

A stronger stroke. Your shoulders share the responsibility of pulling your arms back behind your body, giving you extra power for swimming or rowing.

The Main Move

The barbell military press builds strength and adds size to two of the three sections that make up the deltoids, the most visible muscles of your shoulders. To reduce the risk of injury, use a squat rack and a spotter whenever you perform this classic exercise.

BARBELL MILITARY PRESS

Place a bench in front of a squat rack. Set the barbell in the supports on the rack and step under it. Grab the bar with an overhand grip, your hands slightly more than shoulder-width apart, and hold it so that the middle of the bar is directly above the top of your chest. Then sit on the end of the bench with your feet flat on the floor, keeping your back straight and head facing forward. Press the bar straight over your head. Stop just short of locking your elbows, then slowly lower the bar to your chest.

Perfect Form

Head: Keep your head facing forward and your neck in line with your spine at all times. Tilting your head too far backward or forward can strain the trapezius and neck muscles.

Eyes: Avoid raising your chin to watch the bar as it moves overhead. Stare straight ahead.

Hands: Space them slightly more than shoulder-width apart in an overhand grip (palms facing forward). The bar should rest across your palms so that its weight flows straight through your wrists to your elbows.

Elbows: Keep your elbows pointed down and in line with your upper body at the start of the move. Avoid locking them at the top, so you keep constant tension on your muscles and off your joints.

Wrists: Keep your wrists directly in line with your forearms. This distributes the weight throughout your arms, reducing strain on your joints.

Chest: Lower the bar straight down to the top of your chest. Lowering it too far out in front of you places more stress on your ten-

Challenging Changeups

Dumbbell Press

Assume the same position as for the barbell military press, but use dumbbells instead of a bar. Hold the weights at the sides of your shoulders using an overhand grip, and press them over your head. You'll be able to bring your elbows more directly in line with your shoulders, instead of having to move them forward to avoid hitting your nose with the bar.

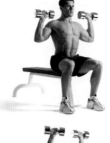

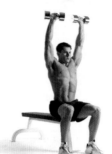

Arnold Press

Named after Governor Schwarzenegger, the Arnold press lengthens the typical range of motion because you start with the weights below your shoulders. Hold a pair of dumbbells in front of you at chest height with an underhand grip. As you push the weights overhead, rotate your arms so that your palms face forward at the top of the movement.

Swiss-Ball Press

Sit on a Swiss ball with your feet flat on the floor. Grab a light barbell (or dumbbells) and hold the weight in front of your chest, hands spaced slightly more than shoulder-width apart. Slowly press the weight over your head until your arms are straight. Using the ball makes it more difficult to stabilize yourself, which not only improves your balance but also makes it harder to rush through the exercise.

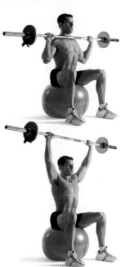

Standing Behind-the-Neck Press

Stand with a barbell resting across the back of your shoulders and hold it with your hands more than shoulder-width apart, palms facing forward. Keeping your back straight and feet flat, press the bar over your head. Lowering the bar behind your neck in this way is a more advanced exercise but may feel more uncomfortable, depending on your body—so listen to it.

---

dons, anterior deltoids, and shoulder joints, increasing your risk of injury.

Lower back: Avoid arching your back and try not to lean. Leaning back not only increases your risk of injury, it places your body at an angle that lets your chest muscles assist with the pressing phase.

Legs: Sit on a bench with your knees bent and your legs apart to help maintain balance during the lift.

Feet: Both feet should be flat on the floor at all times and angled slightly to the sides.

Mix and Max

Go wide. A wider grip emphasizes your shoulders by reducing the amount of effort your triceps can put forth to help perform the move.

Hit "pause." As you lower the bar, stop for a second or two when it's in front of your eyes, then lower it to your chest. This exhausts your muscles faster with less weight than you'd normally need.

Bring it to the back. If lowering the bar to the front feels awkward, try lowering it behind your head—without bending your neck down too far—so that the bar ends up touching the back of your neck.

The Workout

To build a perfect set of shoulders, you need to use a variety of exercises to condition all three of the sections of the deltoid muscles. These six exercises are designed to do just that. After your barbell military-press routine, pick one exercise from each section: A (anterior, or front, deltoids), B (middle, or side, deltoids), and C (posterior, or rear, deltoids). Then create your program using the chart on page 118. You'll design a workout that will strengthen each shoulder from all three sides for maximum development.

BARBELL FRONT RAISE (A)

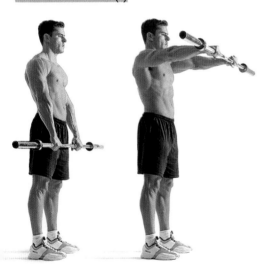

Stand with your feet shoulder-width apart and hold a barbell in front of your thighs. Your hands should be about shoulder-width apart, palms down. Keeping your back and arms straight, slowly raise the bar in an arc in front of you until your arms are parallel to the floor. Pause, then slowly lower the bar until your hands almost touch your thighs.

Get more: Hold an EZ-curl bar at your chest with your palms facing the floor, hands slightly more than shoulder-width apart. Push the bar straight out and away from your body until your arms are straight and parallel to the floor. Pause, then pull the bar back to your chest.

CABLE FRONT RAISE (A)

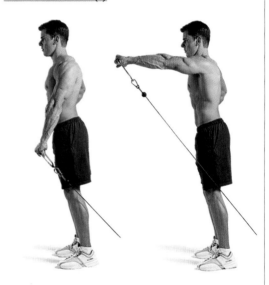

Stand with your back to a low pulley and the handle in your left hand, palm facing behind you. Keeping your back and arm straight, slowly raise your left arm in front of you until it's parallel to the floor. Pause, then slowly lower the handle to the starting position. Finish your repetitions, then repeat with your right hand.

Get more: Attach a straight bar to the low pulley. Stand facing away from the pulley with the bar between your legs, and grab the bar with both hands. With your arms straight and palms facing your thighs, raise the bar out in front of you until your arms are parallel to the floor.

ONE-ARM SIDE RAISE (B)

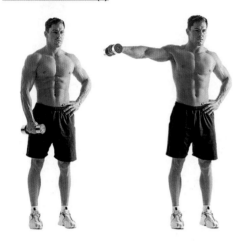

Stand with your feet shoulder-width apart and hold a light dumbbell in your right hand. Your right arm should hang straight at your side, palm facing you; your left hand can rest on your hip. Keeping your right arm straight but your elbow unlocked, slowly raise it to the side until it's parallel to the floor. Pause, then slowly lower the weight to the starting position. After completing the set with your right hand, repeat with your left.

Get more: Instead of lowering the weight all the way to your side, try stopping when your hand is about a foot away from your thigh. Not allowing your arm to hang straight at the bottom of the exercise keeps constant tension on your middle deltoids throughout the lift.

CABLE TWO-ARM RAISE (B)

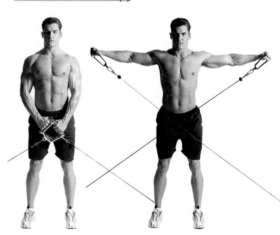

Stand between the weight towers and use your right hand to grab the bottom handle that's to

The Right Workout for You

Build a set of granite-hard shoulders with our easy-to-use chart

YOUR LEVEL	WORK YOUR SHOULDERS	SETS OF EACH EXERCISE	REPETITIONS PER SET	SPEED OF EACH REP	REST BETWEEN SETS
Beginner	Three times a week	1–3	10–15	3–4 seconds up, 3–4 seconds down	30–60 seconds
Intermediate	Twice a week	2–4	8–12	2–3 seconds up, 2–3 seconds down	60–120 seconds
Advanced	Twice a week	3–5	6–8	2 seconds up, 2 seconds down	90–240 seconds

Meet Your Muscles

The deltoid muscles cap your shoulder joints and are made up of three sections—anterior, middle, and posterior.

The anterior (1) and middle (2) deltoids start on the collarbone, while the posterior (3) deltoids start on the scapula (shoulder blade). All three sections come together and attach to the humerus (the upper-arm bone). The main function of your deltoids is to move your arms away from your body, but each set of deltoid fibers has its own role. The anterior section raises your arms in front of your body, the middle section lifts them out to the sides, and the posterior section raises them behind you.

Being located in both the front and back of your body means the deltoids act as secondary movers during numerous exercises. The anterior deltoids assist the pectoral muscles in many chest exercises, while the posterior deltoids assist in many upper-back exercises that involve the teres major, rhomboids, and trapezius.

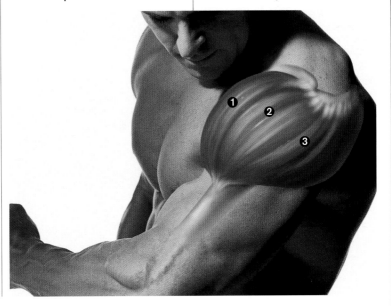

your left. Grab the opposite bottom handle with your left hand and stand with your arms down in front of you, the handles crossing below your waist. Keeping your arms straight but your elbows unlocked, slowly raise your arms out to the sides until they're parallel to the floor and your palms face down. Your body forms a T shape. Pause for a second, then slowly lower your arms to the starting position.

Get more: To better focus on each shoulder independently, stand in the same position but grab only one handle. Do one set, then grab the other handle to work the opposite shoulder.

DUMBBELL BENT-OVER RAISE (C)

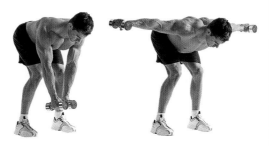

Stand with your knees slightly bent and hold a light weight in each hand. Your arms should hang straight down at your sides, palms facing each other. Bending at the waist, lean forward until your back is flat and as parallel to the floor as possible. Keeping your arms straight and your elbows unlocked, slowly raise the weights out to your sides until your arms are parallel to the floor. Pause for a second, then slowly lower your arms.

Get more: Perform the exercise using an overhand grip. As you raise the weights up and out to your sides, keep your wrists in this position so your palms continue to face backward throughout the motion.

LYING INCLINE-BENCH RAISE (C)

Grab a pair of light dumbbells and lie facedown on a bench that's inclined about 45 degrees. Let your arms hang toward the floor with your palms facing each other. Keeping your arms straight but your elbows unlocked, slowly raise your arms out from your sides until they're parallel to the floor. Pause, then slowly lower the weights to the starting position.

Get more: Exchange the bench for a Swiss ball. Lie facedown with your chest and abs on top of the ball and your arms hanging down at your sides, palms facing in. Maintaining your balance, slowly raise your arms

straight out to your sides in an arc until they're parallel to the floor.

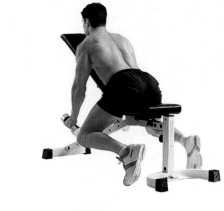

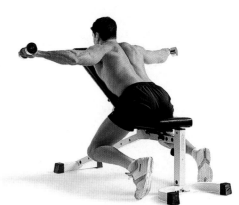

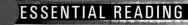

Get a Leg Up

Beef up your
chicken legs with these
muscle-building moves

The Thighs Have It

The quadriceps are the muscles that decide how high you jump, how fast you run, and how good you look in shorts. With all that pressure riding on your quads, it's easy to see why this primary muscle group requires extra attention. You can target the muscles with some isolation exercises, but many leg exercises also recruit help from other muscle groups, both primary (hamstrings) and secondary (glutes, lower back, and calves). Because the quadriceps are stronger than the hamstrings, it's important to exhaust the quads at the start of your leg routine. The smartest workout order: quadriceps first, hamstrings second, calves last.

The Payoff

Better sex. Thrusting forward while propped up on your knees requires a lot of

Meet Your Muscles

Your quadriceps are made up of four individual muscles—hence the name.

The vastus intermedius (1) attaches to and covers much of the front and sides of the femur (your thighbone) but is not visible, as it lies underneath the rectus femoris. The rectus femoris (2) starts at the pelvis and runs down your thigh, in front of the vastus intermedius. The vastus lateralis (3) and vastus medialis (4) begin at the outer and inner sides (respectively) of the top of the femur. All four muscles run down your thigh and converge at the patellar tendon, which attaches along the upper part of the tibia (shinbone).

Together, the four muscles are responsible mainly for extending your knees (straightening your legs), but they also help support the inner and outer sides of your knee joints. Because many of the exercises that target the quadriceps also involve the lower legs, the quads often work in unison with your gastrocnemius and soleus muscles—the main calf muscles.

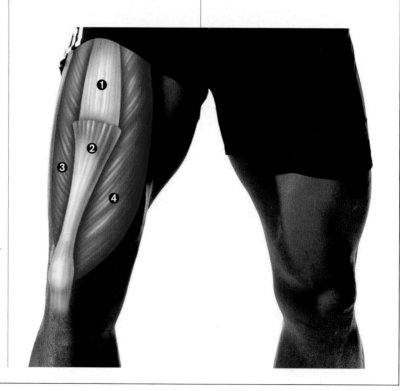

hip flexion and hip extension. Strong quadriceps and hip flexors will help.

Extra stamina. Many sports and activities require constant side-to-side (lateral) movements, which work the quadriceps from the outside of the muscle to the inside. Strengthening your quads will keep them from tiring out and help prevent injury.

Explosive takeoffs. The quadriceps' main job is to extend your knees—in other words, straighten your legs. Training the quads frequently can make it easier to do that job with more force, giving you more power whenever you use your legs to push yourself forward or up.

More stability. Conditioning your quadriceps also strengthens the ligaments and tendons in your legs—critical elements that help support your knees. This in turn makes your knees more stable and less susceptible to injury in the gym or on the playing field.

The Main Move

The squat is the ultimate exercise for developing all the muscles of the lower body, especially the quadriceps.

THE SQUAT

Place a barbell on a squat rack about chest high and stand facing it. Grab the bar with an overhand grip slightly wider than shoulder-width apart, duck underneath it, and rest the bar across the backs of your shoulders. Lift the bar and step back from the rack. With your feet shoulder-width apart and back straight, slowly squat down until your thighs are parallel to the floor. Slowly press yourself back up into a standing position, but don't lock your knees.

Challenging Changeups

Dumbbell Squat

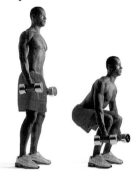

Stand with a dumbbell in each hand, your arms at your sides and your feet shoulder-width apart. Slowly squat until your thighs are parallel to the floor. Using dumbbells instead of a bar may require a stronger grip, but having the weight closer to the floor makes it easier to balance throughout the lift.

Front Squat

Grab the bar with an overhand grip slightly wider than shoulder width and rest it just below your chin. Keep your elbows high and your chest up while you squat. (Your upper arms should be parallel to the floor.) This shifts more of the load off the hamstrings and gluteus muscles and redirects it onto your quadriceps.

Sumo Squat

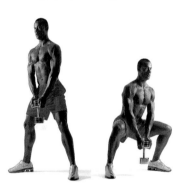

Stand with your feet more than shoulder-width apart, toes pointed out to the sides. Hold a heavy dumbbell with both hands under the top end of the weight and let your arms hang straight down. Squatting in this position helps develop the outside of your legs more specifically.

One-Legged Wall Squat

Stand with your back against a wall, your feet about 18 inches in front of you. Tuck your left foot behind your right calf, then perform a squat on one leg. Do a set, then switch legs. This allows you to focus on building one leg at a time without losing your balance.

Perfect Form

Head: Keep your head facing forward at all times. Moving your head places stress on your neck and trapezius muscles and can cause you to lose your balance.

Eyes: Focus straight ahead and avoid looking down to watch yourself. Looking down or turning your head to either side while you squat makes it more difficult to stay balanced.

Hands: Space them slightly wider than shoulder-width apart, using an overhand grip (palms facing forward). Since the weight of the bar rests across your shoulders, all your hands do is keep the bar from sliding backward.

Shoulders: The bar should rest comfortably across your rear shoulders and trapezius.

Elbows: Your elbows should point straight down, so your forearms are perpendicular to the floor. Pulling the elbows back or shifting them forward places your arms

in an unnatural position that can compromise form.

Wrists: Don't let your wrists bend backward or forward. Keeping them straight in line with your forearms makes it easier to hold the bar in place.

Back: Maintain a straight back throughout the lift. Arching your back prevents the weight from being distributed evenly down to your legs and places unnecessary stress on your lower back and spinal column.

Knees: At the top of the move, straighten your legs, but don't lock your knees. Locking the knees takes the load off your muscles and puts it onto your knee joints. At the bottom of the move, keep your knees directly above your toes; don't let them go past your feet.

Feet: Space your feet shoulder-width apart, with your toes pointing straight ahead, and keep them pressed flat on the floor at all times. Rising up on the balls of

The Right Workout for You
Build impressive quadriceps with our easy-to-use chart

YOUR LEVEL	WORK YOUR QUADRICEPS	SETS OF EACH EXERCISE	REPETITIONS PER SET	SPEED OF EACH REP	REST BETWEEN SETS
Beginner	Three times a week	1–3	10–15	3–4 seconds up, 3–4 seconds down	30–60 seconds
Intermediate	Twice a week	2–4	8–12	2–3 seconds up, 2–3 seconds down	60–120 seconds
Advanced	Twice a week	3–5	6–8	2 seconds up, 2 seconds down	90–240 seconds

your feet can disrupt your balance and make the lift dangerous.

Mix and Max

Vary your stance. By widening your stance a few inches beyond shoulder width, you'll work more of the hamstrings and glutes. Keeping the stance at shoulder width with toes facing out will isolate more of the sides of your thighs.

Go bar hopping. Placing the bar farther down across the rear of your shoulders redistributes the weight backward, which calls in your gluteal and hip muscles to help out. Inching the bar closer to your neck keeps the weight forward, placing more muscle-building stress on your quadriceps.

Adjust your approach. It's not always necessary to squat down until your thighs are parallel to the floor. Lowering yourself halfway or a quarter of the way can still be effective at developing your quadriceps.

The Workout

Building perfect quadriceps means working them through several ranges of motion. That's because your legs can be extended at a variety of angles—toes pointing in or out, feet spread out or drawn in closer. These six exercises provide a mix of isolation exercises and other moves that recruit whatever muscles you want to focus on. After your squat routine, pick one exercise from each section: A (quadriceps), B (quadriceps/hamstrings/glutes), and C (calves). Then build your program using the chart on the opposite page. The end result will be a set of strong, powerful quadriceps.

LEG PRESS (A)

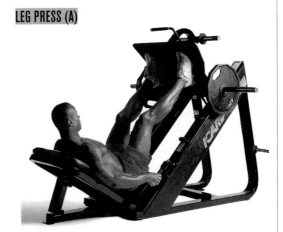

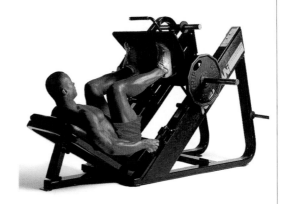

Position yourself in a leg-press machine so that your back and butt are flat against the pads, with your feet hip-width apart on the platform above. Press the weight up until your legs are straight, but keep your knees unlocked. Release the support bar and slowly lower the weight until your legs are bent 90 degrees. Push the weight back up until your legs are straight, knees unlocked.

Get more: Lower the position of your feet on the platform after each set. The lower your feet are on the platform, the better you isolate your quadriceps. The higher your feet, the harder your glutes and hamstrings have to work.

LEG EXTENSION (A)

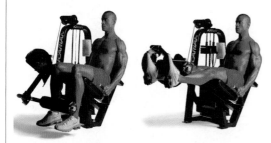

Sit at a leg-extension machine with your ankles tucked under the footpads and your back and buttocks flush against the seat. Slowly extend your legs up and forward until they're straight in front of you, but keep your knees unlocked. Pause, then slowly bend your knees until your legs are back in the starting position.

Get more: Your muscles are stronger during the "eccentric" phase of an exercise—when the weight is being lowered back down. When using a lighter weight for higher repetitions, raise the weight with two legs and lower it with one.

FRONT ANGLED DUMBBELL LUNGE (B)

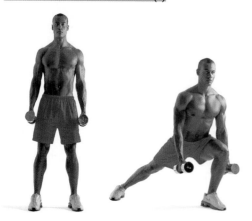

Stand with your feet shoulder-width apart and hold a dumbbell in each hand, arms down at your sides. Step out with your left foot, placing it slightly forward and a few feet to the left. Lean onto your left leg and bend your left knee until your left thigh is almost parallel to the floor, then push back up to the starting position. Repeat the move, this time stepping out with your right foot.

Get more: After each set, return to the starting position with your feet shoulder-width apart, and squat down until your thighs are parallel to the floor. Pause, press yourself back up, and continue with your next set of lunges.

BARBELL LUNGE (B)

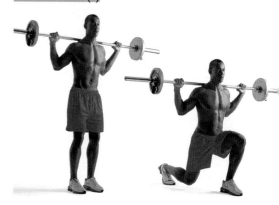

Set a barbell on your shoulders, as you would for a squat, and stand with your feet hip-width apart. Keeping the barbell stationary, take a giant step forward with your left foot and bend your left knee until your left thigh is parallel to the floor and your knee forms a 90-degree angle. Your back should remain straight throughout the exercise. Reverse the motion, stepping back into the starting position. Repeat with your right leg.

Get more: Lunge to the side every other repetition. Keeping your body and toes facing forward, step to your right with your right foot and bend your right knee until your right thigh is almost parallel to the floor. Press yourself back up and repeat with your left leg.

STANDING CALF RAISE (C)

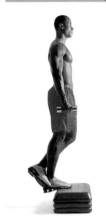

Hold a dumbbell in your right hand and step up onto a stable platform about 6 to 12 inches high. The balls of your feet should rest on the edge of the platform, with your heels hanging off the edge. Place your left hand against a wall for support and tuck your left foot behind your right ankle. (All of your weight should be on the ball of your right foot.) Slowly rise on the toes of your right foot, raising your heel as high as you can. Pause, then slowly lower your heel as far as possible. After a set, switch legs.

Get more: Stand with the balls of both feet on the platform. With your arms out to your sides or holding a pair of light dumbbells, rise on the toes of both feet, then lower yourself. You'll challenge your balance for greater results.

SEATED CALF RAISE (C)

Sit on the edge of a bench and rest the balls of your feet on a step, heels hanging off the edge. Place a weight on your right knee, holding it in place with your hands. Push down on the toes of your right foot to raise your heel as high as you can. Pause, then lower your heel toward the floor as far as you can.

Get more: Placing your feet closer together or farther apart when you do calf

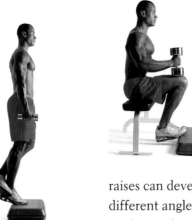

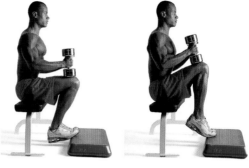

raises can develop your calf muscles from different angles for a more thorough workout. Also, doing the exercise with your shoes off increases your range of motion.

Your Quadriceps' Other Half

Most lifters don't think much about their hamstrings, which are second-class citizens to the quads, the larger, more noticeable thigh muscles. But this group of three muscles at the back of each thigh, running from hip to knee, supports the knees and is critical to balance. Also, the hamstrings, which allow you to bend your knees, are among the most commonly injured leg muscles. Strengthening them properly will help you avoid debilitating injuries. Hamstrings are easy to isolate with leg curls. But many other exercises for this muscle group—the lunge, for example—call your quads and calves into play. To avoid fatigue, we remind you to plan your exercises in this order: quadriceps first, hamstrings second, calves last.

The Payoff

Stronger strides. Your hamstrings pull your heels back toward your butt, while your glutes extend your legs back. Training both can lengthen your stride and offer more power to every push-off.

Better balance. Many hamstring exercises also challenge your stability. The result is a body that can recover quickly when knocked off balance, whether by a bump from a defender or a run on an uneven trail.

Amazing sex. Many women prefer being on top because it lets them lean forward to rub against your pubic bone. Having well-conditioned hamstrings and glutes makes it easier to curl your pelvis forward and up to meet her halfway for more pleasure.

Healthier knees. Your anterior cruciate ligaments (ACLs) rely on your hamstrings to help them stabilize your knees whenever the knees bend while decelerating. Having a strong set of hamstrings can help your ACLs do their job and lower your risk of injury.

The Main Move

The lying hamstring curl is the quintessential isolation exercise for developing and shaping the hamstrings. (Your gym may have a standing or seated leg-curl machine, but the lying leg-curl machine is in most gyms because it's been around the longest.)

LYING HAMSTRING CURL

Lie facedown on a leg-curl machine with your knees hanging off the back edge of the bench. Position your lower legs under the ankle pads so that the undersides of the pads touch your calves just above your ankles. Without moving your upper body, curl your lower legs until the ankle pads are almost touching your gluteus maximus (butt muscles). At the top of the move, contract your glutes for 2 seconds, then lower your legs until they're almost straight.

Perfect Form

Head: Position your head facedown on the pad. Turning your head to the side or tilting it up too far will strain your neck muscles.

Hands: Grab the handles (or the front of the bench) firmly, but resist the urge to use your grip to help you pull yourself forward as you curl.

Chest: Keep your chest flat on the bench. If you feel your chest rising, you're probably using too much weight and/or arching your back to help pull your feet toward your buttocks.

Lower back: Your spine should stay straight throughout the entire exercise.

The Right Workout for You

Build your perfect hamstrings with this checklist

YOUR LEVEL	WORK YOUR HAMSTRINGS	SETS OF EACH EXERCISE	REPETITIONS PER SET	SPEED OF EACH REP	REST BETWEEN SETS
Beginner	Three times a week	1–3	10–15	3–4 seconds up, 3–4 seconds down	30–60 seconds
Intermediate	Twice a week	2–4	8–12	2–3 seconds up, 2–3 seconds down	60–120 seconds
Advanced	Twice a week	3–5	6–8	2 seconds up, 2 seconds down	90–240 seconds

Arching backward only helps curl the weight up and puts unnecessary stress on your lower back.

Hips: Keep your hips flat on the bench. Lifting them takes tension off your hamstrings and places it on your lower back.

Butt: Contract your gluteal muscles at the top of the move (when your heels are close to your butt).

Hamstrings: To build them, keep your thighs together and flat on the bench. Twisting, rotating, or lifting your thighs off the bench cheats your hamstrings by using momentum and other muscles to pull the weight up.

Knees: Your knees should hang just over the edge of the bench. Resting them on the bench makes it easier to hyperextend and strain them as you curl.

Feet: Do not rotate your feet outward or inward, because that can shift some of the effort onto the abductor (outer-thigh) or adductor (inner-thigh) muscles. This can also disrupt your knee alignment, leading to injury.

Ankles: Adjust the roller pads so that the backs of your ankles can tuck underneath them. If the pads rest on your heels, your feet could slip out as you curl the weight up. Having them touch higher on your calves changes the arc of the exercise and robs your hamstrings of work.

Mix and Max

Use two, then one. Muscles can generally handle more weight during the lowering phase of a lift than the lifting phase. Try to curl the weight up with both legs and lower it with one. You'll work your muscles hard during both phases without adjusting the weight.

Blindfold your muscles. Not being able to see your hamstrings can make it hard to focus on them as you exercise. Closing your eyes as you curl can help you visualize the muscles, making it easier to sense whether you're working them thoroughly.

Call in the calves. To involve your calf muscles in the exercise, pull your toes up (toward your knees) at the top of the move (when your heels are near your buttocks).

The Workout

The hamstrings, like the biceps, can resist stress only through a limited range of motion. However, they team up with other muscle groups, such as your quadriceps and glutes, during other exercises that work the legs. These six lifts provide an even mix of isolation exercises and combination moves. After doing the leg curl, pick one exercise from section A (hamstrings) and one from either B (to involve your quads) or C (to involve your glutes). Then select a routine using our chart on page 129. Whichever formula you choose, you'll build the perfect set of hamstrings—even if you'll be the only one who can't see how perfect they are.

DUMBBELL LEG CURL (A)

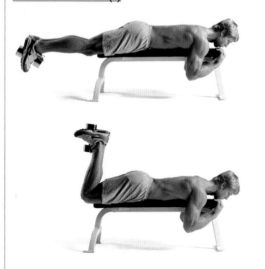

Lie facedown on a flat bench and have your workout partner place a light dumbbell between your feet, with one end of the dumbbell resting on the soles of your shoes. Grab the underside of the bench, but resist the urge to pull yourself forward as you curl. Curl your lower legs back toward your buttocks. Pause, then lower the weight and repeat.

Get more: Try the move lying facedown on a slant board so that your head is above your hips. Because of the angle, you won't be able to completely straighten your legs, which will keep more tension on your hamstrings.

STANDING LEG CURL (A)

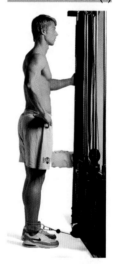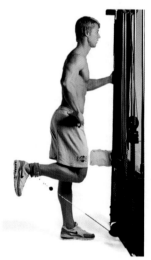

Attach a padded foot strap to a low-cable pulley. Loop your right foot through the strap and stand facing the weight stack, holding the machine for balance. Curl your heel back toward your buttocks. Pause, then lower the foot and repeat. Finish your repetitions with your right leg, then switch the strap to your left foot and repeat.

Get more: Between curls, try keeping your leg straight while raising it behind you. Stop when you feel tension in your hamstrings, then bring your leg forward again.

BARBELL LUNGE (B)

Stand with your feet about 6 inches apart while holding a light barbell on the backs of your shoulders and trapezius. Take a large step forward with your left leg. When your left thigh is parallel to the floor and your knee is directly above your foot, push yourself back to the starting position and repeat the lunge with your right leg.

Get more: After you push yourself back to the starting

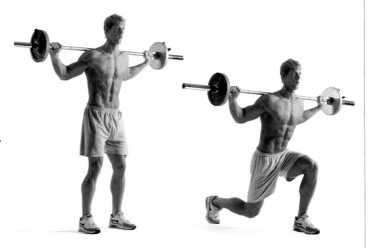

Challenging Changeups

Medicine-Ball Curl

Lie facedown on a flat bench and have a partner place a light medicine ball between your feet. Squeezing your feet together to hold the ball in place also conditions the adductors—located along the insides of your thighs—as you curl.

Stiff-Legged Deadlift

Stand in front of a barbell, your feet hip-width apart and knees unlocked. Bending at the waist, grab the barbell just outside your legs with an overhand grip. Keeping your back flat and legs straight, tighten your glutes and stand back up. Pause, then lower the bar to the floor, keeping your arms straight throughout the move.

Good Morning

Stand with a barbell on your shoulders, your feet shoulder-width apart and knees bent

slightly. Maintain this knee angle throughout the move. Bend forward at the hips as far as you can while keeping your lower back flat or slightly arched. Contract your glutes and push your hips forward to return to the starting position.

Towel Curl

Lie facedown on a mat and bend your lower legs so they form a 45-degree angle. Ask your workout partner to stand behind you and loop a large towel around one of your ankles. Curl your foot up as your partner gently pulls on the towel to apply resistance.

Low-Pulley Cable Curl

Place a mat in front of a low-pulley station and hook an ankle strap to your left leg. Lie facedown on the mat with your feet in front of the weight stack, then slowly curl your left foot toward

your butt. Complete your repetitions, then place the strap on your right leg and repeat. This maneuver makes it easier to isolate your hamstrings one leg at a time so both legs have to work equally hard.

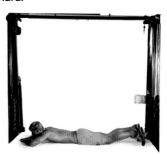

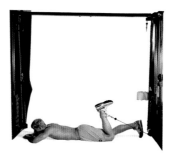

position, step back with the same leg that just lunged forward and bend your legs until your forward leg's thigh is almost parallel to the floor, then return to the starting position. You'll improve your balance even more.

STEP LUNGE (B)

Stand about 3 feet from an exercise step (or a stair) with your feet about 6 inches apart. Hold two dumbbells at your sides, your palms facing in. Keeping your back straight, step forward with your left foot and place it on the step. Lean forward until your left thigh is parallel to the floor. Then push yourself back to the starting position and repeat with your right leg.

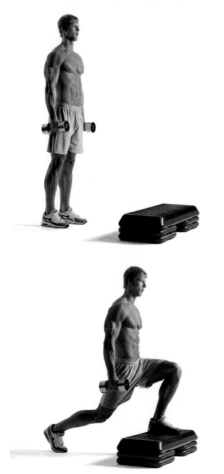

Get more: Start by standing on top of the step with both feet. Step back with your right foot and plant it on the floor. Lunge down until your left thigh is parallel to the floor. Push yourself back onto the step. Repeat, stepping backward with your left foot.

LYING BRIDGE (C)

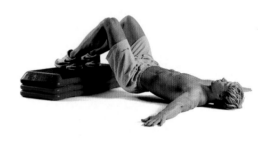

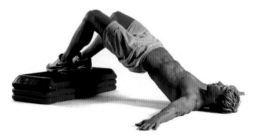

Lie on your back with your knees bent at a 90-degree angle and your heels resting on the edge of a step. Your arms should be flat, out from your sides, palms down for balance. Press down through your heels as you slowly raise your butt, hips, and lower back off the floor until your body forms a straight line from your knees to your shoulders. Pause for 2 seconds, then lower yourself until your butt is about an inch above the floor, and repeat.

Get more: As you grow more comfortable with this exercise, try pressing yourself up with one leg instead of two: Straighten one leg while you press down with the other.

FIRE HYDRANT (C)

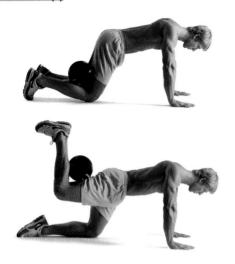

Kneel on all fours on a mat and place a small medicine ball behind your right knee. Squeeze your leg muscles so that the ball stays locked in place. Keeping your back flat and your head down, slowly raise your right leg until the thigh is parallel to the floor. (The leg should form a right angle.) Pause, lower your leg to the starting position, and repeat. Complete the set, then repeat with your left leg.

Get more: Instead of using a bigger ball for more resistance, kneel with your butt facing a low-cable pulley and attach the pulley to one of your ankles. The angle of resistance will change, but you'll still focus on your hamstrings and glutes, using as much weight as you need.

Meet Your Muscles

Located on the backs of your thighs, your hamstrings are made up of three separate muscle groups—the semimembranosus (1), semitendinosus (2), and biceps femoris (3).

The first two muscles start on the ischial tuberosity (just beneath the gluteus maximus, on the pelvic bone) and attach to the medial tibia (the shinbone). The third muscle—the biceps femoris—has two heads. The long head starts on the ischial tuberosity, while the short head attaches to the femur (thighbone). Both heads run down the back of the thigh and insert on the head of the fibula (the smaller bone in the lower leg).

Separately, these three muscles help turn your knees inward and your feet outward. But together, they have two major functions: knee flexion (bending your knees) and hip extension (kicking back a leg). Other muscles assist your hamstrings in performing these two jobs. For instance, whenever you flex your knees, you also use your sartorius gracilis and gastrocnemius muscles. Whenever you extend your hips, your glutes and erector spinae muscles assist in the motion.

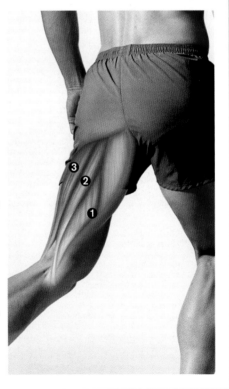

BY MYATT MURPHY

Back on Track

Handle heavy loads
and prevent pain with this
back-to-basics workout

Think Big

If you're looking for big muscles, there are none larger—when it comes to total surface area—than the ones in your upper back. But the upper back is a primary muscle group that requires other, secondary muscle groups, mainly the shoulders and biceps, to assist in exercises. If you work either your shoulders or your arms first, they'll give up on you before you have the chance to thoroughly exhaust your upper-back muscles. The smartest order: upper back first, shoulders second, biceps last.

The Payoff

More pulling power. A stronger upper back not only adds strength to your swimming stroke but helps you pull your body up when climbing, whether up a mountain or a ladder.

A thinner waist. Reshaping your upper back to appear wider at the top helps create a V shape that makes your waistline appear smaller.

A harder throw. Your upper back helps to rotate your upper arms internally, so strengthening it gives you that extra snap of power when you punch or throw.

Perfect posture. Working your back as often as you work your chest helps prevent muscular imbalances that can cause overdeveloped fibers to pull against underutilized ones. That means less risk of posture problems and exercise-related injuries.

The Main Move

The lat pulldown lets you target your upper-back muscles with the least amount of assistance from secondary muscles, so you get more results for your efforts.

PEAK
performance

Lean Back

A slight change in your lat-pulldown form can help you build a stronger back. Since the rhomboids are essential to this move, you'll hit a plateau if yours aren't strong, says Scott Rankin, CSCS.

While sitting at the lat-pulldown station, lean back at a 30-degree angle. With your palms facing forward, pull the bar to your chest. Pause, then return to the starting position. Do two sets of 15 repetitions, using 40 percent less weight than you normally would, to begin your back routine.

LAT PULLDOWN

Attach a long straight bar to the cable of a lat-pulldown station and grab the bar overhead with an overhand grip (palms facing away from you), hands slightly more than shoulder-width apart. Sit with your head and back straight and slowly pull the bar to the top of your chest. Pause, then let the bar rise back above your head—resisting the weight as you go—until your arms are straight with your elbows unlocked.

Perfect Form

Head: Avoid tilting your head back to look up at the bar. This places excessive stress on your neck muscles.

Neck: Never bring the bar down behind your neck. This deviation limits the range of motion and causes your shoulders to rotate backward, putting excessive stress on weaker tendons and increasing your risk of developing shoulder tendinitis.

Arms: Resist the weight as the bar pulls your arms straight over your head, and keep your elbows unlocked.

Elbows: At the bottom of the move—with the bar pulled down to your chest—your elbows should be pointing down and slightly behind you.

Wrists: Keep your wrists in line with your forearms at all times. Bending them forward or backward as you pull the bar down places unnecessary stress on your wrists and forearms, causing them to tire before your back muscles and become more susceptible to injury.

Hands: Grab the bar with an overhand grip, with your thumbs wrapped around the bar. Your hands should be spaced slightly more than shoulder-width apart.

Chest: Lower the bar to the top of your chest instead of behind your neck. This makes it impossible to lean forward and prevents shoulder impingement.

Lower back: As you pull the bar down to your chest, it's fine to lean back slightly, but keep your back flat throughout the exercise. Arching backward too far or fast to help draw the bar down uses more momentum than muscle.

Legs: Adjust the leg pads so that your knees are tucked firmly underneath.

Feet: Both feet should be flat on the floor at all times and angled to the sides for better balance.

Mix and Max

Move your hands. Perform one set with your hands shoulder-width apart, then widen or narrow the space between your hands by an inch or two for each remaining set. Changing your hand spacing changes the angle of the exercise and its effect on the muscles, so you can work the muscles several ways with the same exercise.

Grip so you don't slip. If your biceps tire before your back muscles, try wrapping your thumbs on the same side of the bar as your fingers so that your hands "hook" the bar instead of encircling it. This variation makes it harder for the forearms to get in-

The Right Workout for You

Build a wider, stronger upper back with our easy checklist

YOUR LEVEL	WORK YOUR UPPER BACK	SETS OF EACH EXERCISE	REPETITIONS PER SET	SPEED OF EACH REP	REST BETWEEN SETS
Beginner	Three times a week	1–3	12–15	3-4 seconds up, 3-4 seconds down	30-60 seconds
Intermediate	Twice a week	2–4	8–12	2-3 seconds up, 2-3 seconds down	60-120 seconds
Advanced	Twice a week	3–5	8–12	2-3 seconds up, 2-3 seconds down	90-240 seconds

Meet Your Muscles

Your upper back is made up of several muscle groups—the latissimus dorsi and the trapezius being the most impressive.

The latissimus dorsi (1), the largest muscles of the back, are a set of fan-shaped muscles that start at the upper end of the humerus (upper-arm bone) and run down to attach low on the vertebral column and pelvic girdle. Located on both sides of the body, they serve primarily to pull the arm down. They can also pull the body up toward the arm. For each of these tasks, the lats get assistance from the teres major—a muscle that runs from the outer edge of the scapula (shoulder blade) to the humerus.

The trapezius muscles (2) are long, triangle-shaped muscles that start at the base of the skull and attach to the backs of the collarbones and scapulae. They have several jobs, including scapular elevation (shrugging your arms up), scapular depression (pulling the shoulder blades down), and scapular adduction (pulling the shoulder blades together). Beneath the trapezius lie the rhomboids, muscles that also assist with scapular adduction.

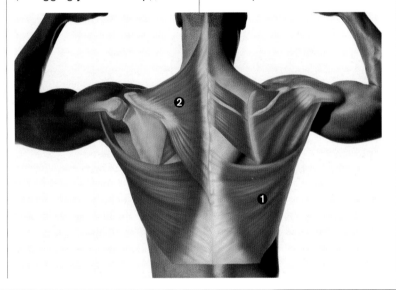

volved, focusing more of your efforts on your back.

Pin your shoulders. Gently pull your shoulder blades down to initiate the move, then squeeze them together at the bottom. This small tweak engages more muscle fibers to assist during the movement.

The Workout

Your upper back is home to the body's largest muscle group—the latissimus dorsi, or lats. Because of the lats' size and various at-tachments, they need to be challenged from several angles. The trapezius muscles (traps) lend support during any exercise that involves the lats, but they can still be isolated. These six moves target your lats and traps with a variety of positions. After your lat-pull-down routine, pick one or two exercises from section A (latissimus dorsi and middle trapezius) and one from B (upper trapezius). Build your program using the chart on the opposite page. You'll hit your back muscles equally through the widest variety of angles.

BENT-OVER ROW (A)

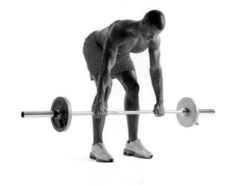

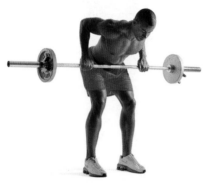

Stand with a barbell on the floor in front of you, with your feet shoulder-width apart and your knees slightly bent. Bend forward at the waist and push your hips back a bit until your torso is almost parallel to the floor. (Your arms should hang straight down.) Lift the bar off the floor using an overhand grip, hands slightly more than shoulder-width apart. Keeping your back and legs still, slowly pull the bar up until it touches your chest just below your pectoral muscles. Pause, then slowly lower the bar.

Get more: Try using a set of dumbbells instead of a bar so you can raise the weights farther. You may have to use less weight, but by pulling your arms back through a greater range of motion, you'll activate more muscle fibers.

DUMBBELL PULLOVER (A)

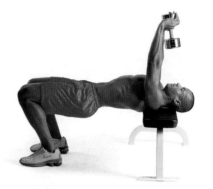

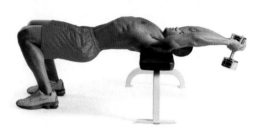

Grab a light dumbbell and rest your shoulders and upper back on a bench. Your head should hang off one side of the bench, while your body is supported on the opposite side by your legs and feet. Wrapping your thumbs and forefingers in a diamond shape around the handle, use both hands to hold the weight vertically over your head. Keeping your elbows slightly bent, slowly lower the weight backward in an arc over your head until you feel a slight stretch in your sides and your upper arms are in line with your head. Pause, then slowly pull the weight back over your chest.

Get more: You can do the same exercise by lying flat on the bench instead of across it. Using the bench in this way makes it easier to hold one weight with both hands or to grab a pair of dumbbells—palms facing each other—and perform the same motion.

ONE-ARM ROW (A)

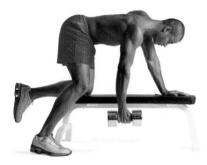

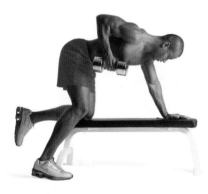

Hold a dumbbell in your right hand. Place your left hand and knee on an exercise bench and let your right arm hang straight down or just in front of your shoulder, your palm facing the bench. Pull the dumbbell up, keeping it close to your body, until it reaches your chest. Lower it until your arm is straight and finish the set. Switch the weight to your left hand, place your right hand and knee on the bench, and repeat.

Get more: Try rotating your wrist inward 180 degrees as you lower the dumbbell so that your palm faces away from the bench when your arm is straight. This helps bring together the scapulae, working the back through a fuller range of motion, for added strength and size.

Challenging Changeups

Pullup

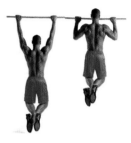

This classic exercise lets you perform the same movement as the lat pulldown, without anything more than a bar and your body weight. Grab a chinup bar with your hands slightly more than shoulder-width apart, palms facing away from you. Hang with your arms straight and your elbows unlocked. Pull yourself up until your chest is even with the bar, then lower yourself back down.

Parallel-Grip Pulldown

Attach a parallel-grip bar to the cable of a lat-pulldown station and grab the handles so that your palms are facing each other. Keeping your head and back straight, slowly pull the bar down until it touches the top of your chest. By positioning your hands closer in and facing each other, you work more muscle fibers in the middle of your upper back.

One-Arm Pulldown

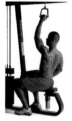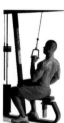

Attach a stirrup handle to the cable of a lat-pulldown station and grab it with your left hand, palm facing in. Slowly pull the handle down until it touches the left side of your chest, then return to the starting position. After you complete a set, repeat with your right hand. This works your back through a greater range of motion than using a bar, which eventually hits your chest and prevents you from pulling your hands back any farther.

Reverse-Grip Pulldown

Try grabbing the straight bar at the lat-pulldown station with an underhand grip. This variation builds your upper-back muscles while letting the biceps help curl the bar at the bottom of the move. Also, the position forces the forearms, wrists, and hands to work harder than they have to in most back exercises, helping you develop a stronger grip at the same time.

WIDE-GRIP SEATED ROW (A)

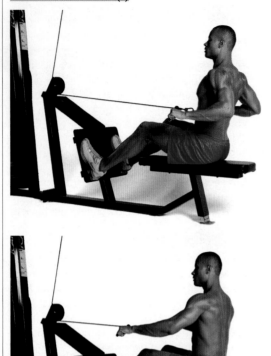

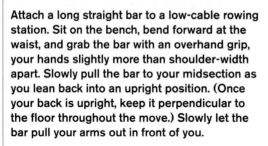

UPRIGHT ROW (B)

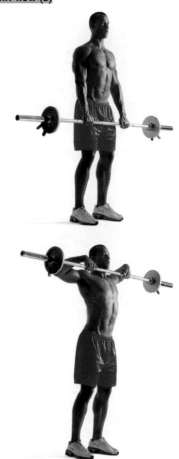

Attach a long straight bar to a low-cable rowing station. Sit on the bench, bend forward at the waist, and grab the bar with an overhand grip, your hands slightly more than shoulder-width apart. Slowly pull the bar to your midsection as you lean back into an upright position. (Once your back is upright, keep it perpendicular to the floor throughout the move.) Slowly let the bar pull your arms out in front of you.

Get more: Bend forward at your waist as you let the bar slowly pull your arms out in front of you. This adjustment lengthens the range of motion and works more of your lower-back muscles.

Stand holding a barbell with an overhand grip, your hands shoulder-width apart and arms hanging straight in front of you so the bar rests against your thighs. Keeping your back straight, slowly lift the bar, keeping it close to your body, until it's just under your chin. Pause, then slowly lower the bar.

Get more: Trade in your barbell for a pair of dumbbells to make the exercise easier on your wrists. Grab the dumbbells with an overhand grip, hands shoulder-width apart. Raise the weights straight up and close to your body until they reach your chest, then lower them.

SEATED SHRUG (B)

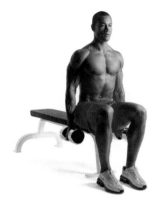

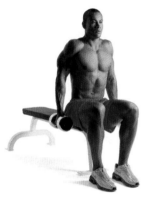

Sit on the end of a bench, with a dumbbell in each hand. Your arms should be hanging at your sides, palms facing each other. With your back straight and your head facing forward, slowly raise your shoulders as high as you can toward your ears. Be careful not to bend your arms as you go or you'll remove tension from the trapezius muscles. Pause, then slowly lower your shoulders until your arms hang down as far as possible.

Get more: Try the exercise one arm at a time. This lets you focus on each side for better development and makes it more difficult to use momentum to cheat the weight up.

Lower Expectations

The lower back is a muscle group that no one thinks about until it hurts. But here's a truth you can't ignore: The lower back is a vital player in your quest for overall health and strength. You must concentrate on it if you want the rest of your muscles to grow bigger and stronger in the safest and fastest way. The lower back works in unison with the abdominals to maintain your posture—essential for any exercise that requires a straight back. Work your lower back too soon, though, and it'll be too weak to help support you later, when you're exercising other muscle groups. The smartest order: upper back first, lower back last.

The Payoff

Extra strength. Pulling, swinging, and throwing hard all rely on transferred power that comes from twisting your torso. Building up your lower-back muscles reinforces your core so your waist can deliver more twisting power when you need it.

Bigger muscles. The stronger your lower-back muscles are, the more supportive they'll be during exercises that work other muscles. You'll see better results with less risk of injury from improper posture.

More energy. A stronger spine allows you to eliminate unnecessary steps or motions as you move. A healthy lower back can help your body perform tasks with less effort and fatigue.

A flatter stomach. Standing straight takes strong, resilient muscles along the spine and

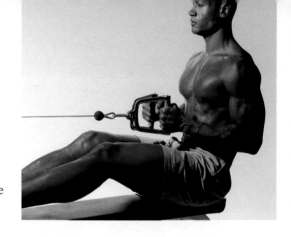

throughout the lower back. The stronger these muscles are, the better they'll minimize the slouching that pushes your stomach out.

The Main Move

The seated row is ideal for developing the entire back. In this version, you bend at the waist to isolate muscles of the lower back.

Sit at a rowing machine (or a low-pulley cable) with your feet flat on the footrests and knees slightly bent. Bending at the waist, lean forward and grasp the handles of a parallel-grip bar, palms facing each other. Slowly draw the handles toward your midsection while leaning back until your torso is perpendicular to the floor. The handles should touch you just below your chest as you become upright. Pause, then slowly lean forward from the waist, straightening your arms, until you return to the starting position.

Perfect Form

Head: Keep your head and neck in line with your spine throughout the move. Turning or raising your head can strain neck muscles that are already contracted during the exercise.

Eyes: Focus on the handles when they're in front of you, but avoid tucking your chin to watch them move toward your midsection. Instead, stare straight ahead.

Arms: Let the weight pull your arms out in front of you at the start of the move. As you begin to lean back, slowly bend your arms to help draw the handles toward your body.

Elbows: At the start of the exercise, keep your elbows unlocked. As you pull the handles toward your midsection, concentrate on drawing your elbows straight back behind you.

The Right Workout for You

Build the perfect lower back with our easy-to-use chart

YOUR LEVEL	WORK YOUR LOWER BACK	SETS OF EACH EXERCISE	REPETITIONS PER SET	SPEED OF EACH REP	REST BETWEEN SETS
Beginner	Three times a week	1–3	12–15	3–4 seconds up, 3–4 seconds down	30–60 seconds
Intermediate	Twice a week	2–4	8–12	2–3 seconds up, 2–3 seconds down	60–120 seconds
Advanced	Twice a week	3–5	8–12	2–3 seconds up, 2–3 seconds down	90–240 seconds

Meet Your Muscles

The erector spinae—or spinal erectors—is a deep-muscle group running along both sides of the spinal column, from the iliac crest (the back of the pelvis) to the ribs, vertebrae, and skull. Each erector is made up of three separate vertical columns of muscle—the iliocostalis (1; farthest from the spine); longissimus (2; in the middle); and spinalis (3; closest to the spine). Each of these three muscles divides into three segments, each named for one of four locations along the spinal column: the capitis (nearest the skull), cervicis (in the neck), thoracis (in the mid-back), or lumborum (in the lower back).

Together, they work to extend the spine (straightening it after it's been flexed forward) and bend it posteriorly (arching your back). They also help support your spinal column and assist with the extension and rotation of your head.

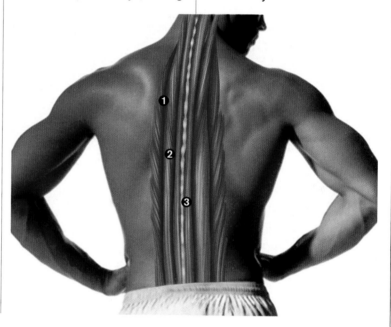

Wrists: Don't let your wrists bend in as you pull, or your forearm muscles could give out before your back does. Keeping them straight will distribute the weight throughout your arms so more of the effort focuses on your back.

Hands: Grab the handles firmly with both hands, palms facing in.

Abs: Keep them tight. The handles should end up directly in front of your upper abdomen, right below your chest. If you feel your shoulder blades rise as you pull, you've pulled the handles too high.

Lower back: Your lower back should remain as flat as possible. Hunching forward places unnecessary stress on your lower back and spinal column. If you find it difficult to perform the move without hunching, you're probably using too much weight.

Butt: Sit flat on the bench so your body is even with the pulley in front of you. Sitting too much to one side can alter the angle of the exercise and make it more difficult to keep your wrists in line with your forearms.

Legs: Sit with your legs slightly bent, knees unlocked, and hold them in this position throughout the move. Bending and straightening your legs lets your quadriceps help pull the weight, cheating your back muscles out of some of the stress.

Feet: Both feet should be pressed flat on the platform in front of you at all times. If the footrest is a rounded bar that doesn't accommodate your entire foot, place your heels on the bar. Raising either foot as you perform the move disrupts your balance and places excessive stress on the knee of the leg that's still in place.

Mix and Max

No-slip grip. If your biceps tire out before your back muscles do, try wrapping your thumbs on the same side as your fingers. This makes it harder for the biceps to get involved.

Less arms, more back. Instead of using your arms to pull the weight toward your midsection, use less weight than normal and keep your arms straight—elbows unlocked—throughout the move. This keeps your upper back and biceps from helping out, so you isolate the muscles in your lower back.

Aim higher. Instead of pulling the handles toward your stomach, pull them toward the middle of your chest. This tweak isolates more of your trapezius, latissimus dorsi, and rhomboid muscles to add extra power to your stroke, swing, or serve.

The Workout

Okay, working your lower back isn't exciting, but it's crucial to developing support for your body in countless other exercises.

These six exercises may seem similar, but the lower back doesn't require much movement to stimulate the muscles. After performing the seated row, pick one exercise from section A (lower back and glutes) and one from either B (if you're in a gym) or C (if you don't have access to equipment). Then build your program using the chart on page 142. Whichever plan you design, your lower back will be stronger and more reliable whenever the rest of your muscles need it.

STIFF-LEGGED DUMBBELL DEADLIFT (A)

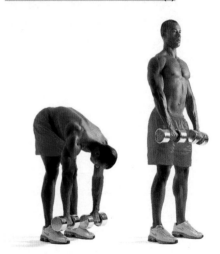

Stand with a pair of dumbbells on the floor in front of you, with your feet hip-width apart and your knees unlocked. Bending at the waist, reach down and grab the dumbbells so they're near your ankles and your palms face your feet. Keeping your back flat and legs straight (knees still unlocked), slowly raise yourself back up into a standing position, keeping your arms straight. Pause, then lower the weights back to the floor.

Get more: Leave the dumbbells on the floor and lift your left foot an inch. Slowly raise yourself into a standing position, then lower yourself back down, keeping your back flat and your knees at the same angle. Touch the weights, then repeat the move with your right foot raised.

INCLINE KICKBACK (A)

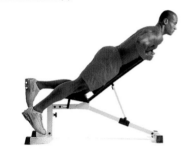

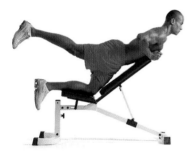

Place your left knee on the end of a bench set at 30 to 45 degrees and put your chest against the pad. Grab the sides of the bench for support, then straighten your right leg, keeping the knee slightly bent. Slowly raise your right leg as high as you comfortably can. Pause, then lower your leg, keeping your foot off the floor to maintain tension on your muscles. Finish your reps, then switch positions to work the left side.

Get more: To raise your leg against more resistance, wrap exercise tubing around the ankle of the working leg and tie the other end to either the bottom of the bench or a dumbbell placed in front of the bench.

Challenging Changeups

Wide-Grip Seated Row

Attach a straight bar to the cable and grab the bar with your hands more than shoulder-width apart, palms down. Slowly draw the bar toward your abs while leaning back until your torso is perpendicular to the floor. This works more of the muscles along the sides of your back (latissimus dorsi), adding width to your back.

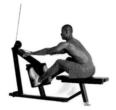 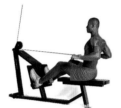

Rope-Handle Seated Row

Attach a rope to the cable and grab an end with each hand, palms facing each other (thumbs up). Doing the seated row this way gives you more maneuverability at your wrists and works the muscles of your hands and forearms.

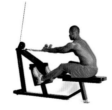 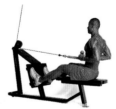

Single-Arm Cable Row

Attach a single handle and grab it with your left hand. Perform the seated row with one hand. This teaches your lower back to work with other muscles to help maintain your balance.

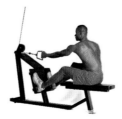 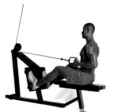

HYPEREXTENSION (B)

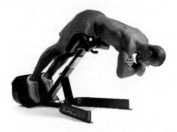

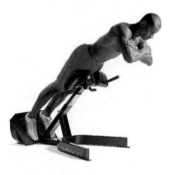

BENCH TWIST (B)

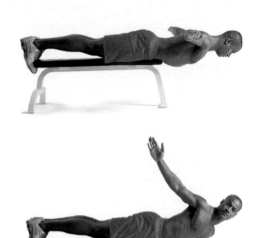

Lie across a hyperextension bench, tucking your ankles securely behind the footpads. Your thighs should lie flat against the wide pad in the front, leaving you enough room to bend at the waist without restriction. Fold your arms and slowly bend forward at the waist as far as you comfortably can, keeping your back flat. Slowly raise your torso until your upper body is slightly higher than parallel to the floor. Pause, then slowly lower yourself to the starting position.

Get more: Switch your arm position by either extending your arms out to the sides or placing your hands by your head, lightly touching your ears. At the top of the movement, twist your body to the left. Lower yourself, then repeat, this time twisting to your right.

Lie facedown on an exercise bench with your torso hanging off the end of the bench. Your hips should be touching the edge of the bench so you can bend at the waist. Raise your torso until your body is perfectly straight, and extend your arms out to the sides. Slowly turn your torso to the left. Pause, then slowly turn to the right.

Get more: Instead of extending your arms out from your sides, hold a light weight plate or medicine ball across your chest.

LYING HYPEREXTENSION (C)

Lie facedown with your arms behind you and your fingers interlaced behind your lower back. Raise your arms behind you, pressing your knuckles toward your feet, then slowly raise your chest off the floor as high as you comfortably can. (Your feet and legs should stay on the floor.) Hold this position for a few seconds, then lower your chest.

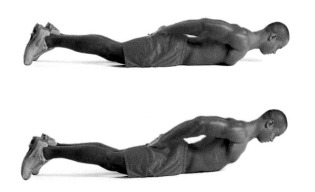

Get more: Lie facedown on a Swiss ball—with just your abs and chest touching—and place your hands alongside your ears. Being positioned on the ball allows you to work your back through a greater range of motion because you can lower your upper body past parallel to the floor.

DRY-LAND SWIMMING (C)

Lie facedown with your arms straight in front of you and your legs straight. Keeping your head facing the floor, simultaneously raise your arms and legs about 6 to 8 inches off the floor. Slowly kick your legs up and down while drawing your arms out to the sides and back in behind you. Continue for as many repetitions as possible.

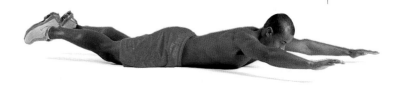

Get more: Every time you sweep your arms behind you, bring your legs back together, keeping them raised off the floor, and hold this position for 2 seconds.

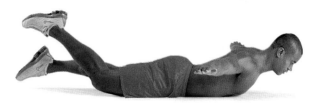

Training Tips

TRY A DIFFERENT APPROACH

Q **I'm curling like a madman, but my biceps have stopped growing. What's up with that?**

H.G., ABILENE, TEXAS

A Our solution: Stop curling for 4 weeks. And try this self-test: Stand with natural posture and look at your hand position. Your arms are probably rotated so that your palms are slightly in front of and facing your body. This means your trapezius and rhom-

boids—back muscles that stabilize your arms when you do curls—aren't strong enough to handle the heavy weights needed to grow your biceps. The following exercise strengthens the support mechanism of the upper spine "so you can handle greater loads when you return to curling," says Alwyn Cosgrove, CSCS, owner of Results Fitness Training in Santa Clarita, California. Do two sets of 10 to 15 repetitions every 4 days.

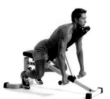 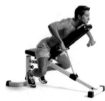

Set an incline bench at a 45-degree angle. Grab a pair of light (5- to 10-pound) dumbbells with an overhand grip and lie with your chest against the pad. Let your arms hang straight down from your shoulders.

Move your upper arms perpendicular to your body and lift them as high as you can by bending your elbows and squeezing your shoulder blades together.

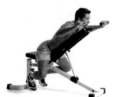 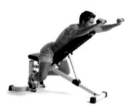

Then, without changing the position of your upper arms, raise your forearms by rotating them upward until they're in line with your body.

Keeping your shoulder blades pulled together, press the weights straight over your head. Reverse the movement and return to the starting position.

SHOULDERS ABOVE

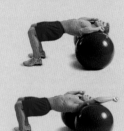

Get on the Ball

Two Swiss balls can pump up your shoulders in no time. Try this shoulder-press variation from Mike Mejia, MS, CSCS.

Position two small Swiss balls together and lie back on them so that your head is between, but not resting on, them. Your upper back and shoulders should rest on the balls. Keep your knees bent and your hips raised so your body looks like a table. Bend your elbows 90 degrees.

With your abs tight, straighten one arm over your head. (Try to keep that shoulder in contact with the ball.) Bring your arm back down, then straighten your other arm. "Both shoulders, especially the shoulder of the straight arm, have to work hard to stabilize you," says Mejia. Try for two sets of 8 to 10 reps.

Balancing Act

Reduce your chance of injury by doing pullups to balance the strength in your upper body. This exercise is crucial to the "shoulder girdle," the musculature that connects your shoulders, chest, and upper

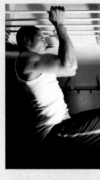

back. Australian researchers reporting in the *Journal of Strength and Conditioning Research* say that many athletes can press 15 percent more weight than they can pull. Study author Robert Newton, PhD, suggests this self-test: Do one set of as many pullups (or lat pull-downs) as you can. On another day, bench-press your body weight (or your lat-pull-down weight) to fatigue. If the front and rear of your shoulders are balanced, you should be able to do about the same number of repetitions of each move.

I hear squats are great for your legs, but they hurt my back. What exercise can replace the squat?

O.F., MUNCIE, INDIANA

First, get your back checked out. A licensed physical therapist can help you keep it from hurting in the future. In the short term, any combination of front squats, split squats, lunges, and stepups should place less pressure on your back. To do a split squat, hold dumbbells at your sides and place one foot for-

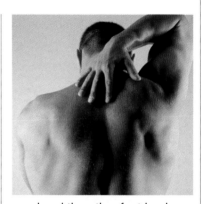

ward and the other foot back so your feet are in a split stance. Drop your hips straight down by bending your knees. (Keep your chest up and don't let your front knee slide forward.) Then press yourself back up.

A Bicycle Built for Six

The bicycle maneuver is a famously efficient abdominal exercise—pumping your legs while rotating your torso works the obliques and your entire six-pack. This Swiss-ball variation from Scott Rankin, CSCS, is even more challenging.

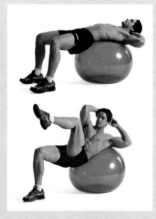

Lie on your back on a Swiss ball, with your knees bent at 90 degrees, your feet flat, and your hands behind your ears. Keeping your right foot planted, lift your left foot off the floor and bring it toward you as you curl your torso up and to the left so your right elbow meets your left knee. Do 12 repetitions. Then plant your left foot on the floor and curl toward your right knee for another 12 reps.

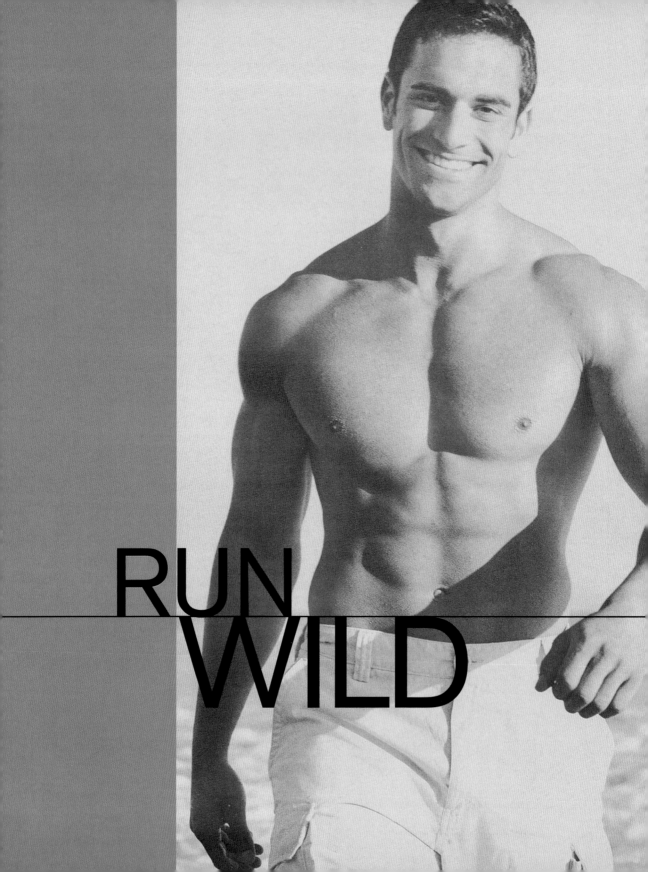

RUN
WILD

In your busy life you do a lot of running—you run to the store, the bank, the dry cleaner. And it probably seems like you're constantly running on empty, what with those measly 6.9 hours of sleep you get on average each night. Sometimes you feel like you just want to run away from it all.

Well, here's your chance—your license to return to simpler days. The days when "running around" meant chasing girls on the playground, not running errand after errand.

Our tips on taking to the trails will give you the motivation and confidence to step off the treadmill, get outside, and put the fun back into running. We'll show you how to add miles to your runs, prevent injuries with advice from top docs, and ease muscle soreness after those particularly tough runs. Ready to take your running to the next level? Prepare for your first half-marathon with our 12-week training program. If you're already a serious runner, try our cross-training tips and discover the perfect speed for your training runs, so that on race day you'll be leading the pack.

And, most important, start looking forward to that hour or so each day when you actually do get to run away from it all.

BY MATT FITZGERALD

Halfway There

**For a bigger fitness challenge—
and sheer fat-burning power—
step up to the half-marathon**

Watching a distance race can be irritating *and* inspiring. Fit guys and hot women, all moving too fast and looking a bit too self-satisfied. And yeah, you'd like to be out there with them. That's the inspiring part.

But maybe you've got a gut. Or you're out of shape, or you've never run that far in your life. Listen: Those aren't reasons you can't run a race. Those are reasons you should.

And you might as well make it an impressive distance, like the half-marathon. It's serious running with serious benefits. By the time you actually run the 13.1-mile race later this year—and it's going to happen—you'll have a rock-solid midsection, looser pants, and a guilt-free appetite. You may have to field flattering questions from women and vague resentment from softer friends, but you can handle that.

Signing up for a "half"—you might as well start using runners' shorthand—is a *venti* jolt of motivation. Half-marathons are numerous now, and crowded.

A popular race is good—all those people mean more support. A half is a fun challenge that requires much less preparation than a full marathon. And if you mumble when you tell them about it, people might think you did run a marathon.

There's a trick to the training: Limit your running. Cross-training is crucial for success. I've written a book, *Runner's World Guide to Cross-Training* (Rodale), which was based on my foray into triathlons after 15 years as a runner. Going in, I figured my training as a runner would make me a respectable swimmer and bicyclist. But I had it backward—the swimming and biking (and weight training) made me a faster, stronger runner, even though I was running less.

That's the key to a new you this year. By mixing running with some nonimpact cardio and functional strength training, you'll avoid boredom and sidestep injuries. You'll add lean muscle and simultaneously roast away your gut and build endurance. And you'll be out there with the crowd, striding with the envied instead of standing with the envious. Here's how you'll do it.

The Long Run

You can build the endurance you need to run a successful half-marathon on a foundation of just three runs a week. That's right, three times a week. Do one designated longer run each week, increasing the distance each time, but every third or fourth week, cut back a bit for recovery. Work your way up to a 12-mile run about a week before race day.

The 12-week training schedule on page 154 assumes you can already run 4 miles comfortably. If you haven't been running at all lately, take a few weeks to work up to 4 miles, then jump into the schedule.

The Hard Run

A second weekly run should be a high-intensity workout, such as a set of short intervals. These workouts will increase your efficiency, allowing you to run faster using less energy. Start with an easy 5- to 10-minute warmup. Then do a series of four to six hard runs lasting 30 to 90 seconds each and separated by easy jogs of the same duration. Cool down with another 5 to 10 minutes of easy jogging. The schedule shows a sensible progression for interval training.

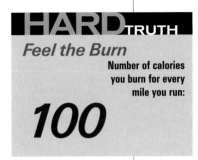

HARD TRUTH

Feel the Burn

Number of calories you burn for every mile you run:

100

The Regular Run

Your third run each week should be moderate in length (4 to 6 miles) and intensity (maintain a steady effort level; think 6 or 7 on a scale of 1 to 10).

The Cross-Training

Once a week, do a nonimpact cardio workout such as bicycling. Most elite runners do this to supplement their cardiovascular fitness while limiting the pounding they inflict on their legs. These workouts should last 20 to 40 minutes at an effort level of 6 or 7.

Elliptical training, deepwater running, bicycling (stationary or outdoors), inline skating, and stairclimbing all provide good crossover benefits for running.

The Lifting

Running is a strength sport—really. Strong core muscles and overall muscle balance increase your joint stability and reduce the likelihood of injuries. Powerful muscles also allow you to take longer, quicker strides. Do two strength sessions per week, focusing on exercises that build leg power and core-muscle strength. Here are three good ones. Do two or three sets of each, plus any others you care to throw in for vanity's sake.

12-Week Half-Marathon Training Plan

	SUNDAY	MONDAY	TUESDAY	WEDNESDAY	THURSDAY	FRIDAY	SATURDAY
Week 1	4-mile run	Rest	Strength workout	Intervals (4 × 30 seconds)	Strength workout	4-mile run	Nonimpact cardio workout
Week 2	5-mile run	Rest	Strength workout	Intervals (5 × 30 seconds)	Strength workout	4-mile run	Nonimpact cardio workout
Week 3	6-mile run	Rest	Strength workout	Intervals (6 × 30 seconds)	Strength workout	4-mile run	Nonimpact cardio workout
Week 4 (recovery)	5-mile run	Rest	Strength workout	Intervals (5 × 30 seconds)	Strength workout	4-mile run	Nonimpact cardio workout
Week 5	7-mile run	Rest	Strength workout	Intervals (4 × 60 seconds)	Strength workout	5-mile run	Nonimpact cardio workout
Week 6	8-mile run	Rest	Strength workout	Intervals (5 × 60 seconds)	Strength workout	5-mile run	Nonimpact cardio workout
Week 7	9-mile run	Rest	Strength workout	Intervals (6 × 60 seconds)	Strength workout	5-mile run	Nonimpact cardio workout
Week 8 (recovery)	7-mile run	Rest	Strength workout	Intervals (5 × 60 seconds)	Strength workout	5-mile run	Nonimpact cardio workout
Week 9	9-mile run	Rest	Strength workout	Intervals (4 × 90 seconds)	Strength workout	6-mile run	Nonimpact cardio workout
Week 10	10-mile run	Rest	Strength workout	Intervals (5 × 90 seconds)	Strength workout	6-mile run	Nonimpact cardio workout
Week 11	11-mile run	Rest	Strength workout	Intervals (6 × 90 seconds)	Strength workout	6-mile run	Nonimpact cardio workout
Week 12	12-mile run	Rest	Strength workout	4-mile run	Nonimpact cardio workout	Rest	Half-marathon race day

CLOCK LUNGE

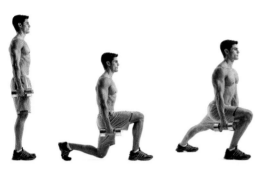

Take a moderately large step forward (to 12 o'-clock) with your right leg and dip down until your left knee almost touches the floor. Keep your torso stable. Now thrust back to the starting position. Lunge four more times: to 1 o'clock, 3 o'clock, 5 o'clock, and 6 o'clock, returning to the starting position after each lunge. Now, with your left leg, lunge to 12, 11, 9, 7, and 6 o'clock. (To make this exercise more challenging, hold dumbbells at your sides or rest a barbell on your shoulders.)

WOOD CHOP

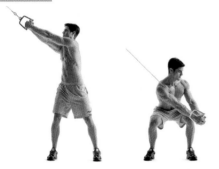

Attach a handle to a high-pulley cable (or a resistance band to the top of a door). Stand in a wide stance with your right side facing the attachment and most of your weight on your right foot. Rotate your torso to the right so you're facing the attachment, and grasp the handle in both hands, arms extended. Using both arms, pull the handle down and across your body, at the same time bending and turning your torso. Continue until the handle is next to your left ankle. Return smoothly to the starting position. Complete 10 repetitions, then switch sides.

REVERSE WOOD CHOP

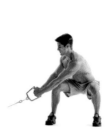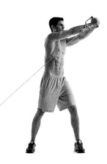

Perform the wood chop in reverse: Attach a handle to a low pulley. Pull it across your body from low to high.

Keep Your Wheels Turning

Increasing mileage increases your chances of injury. "If you can't run on back-to-back days, there's something wrong," says John F. Connors, DPM, a podiatric physician who treats world-class runners. Watch for pains that get worse with each workout and persistent swelling in the knees, ankles, or feet. For prevention:

Go soft. Hard, uneven surfaces compound your risk of nagging injuries like shinsplints. Find surfaces like grass, dirt, wood chips, or a track.

Drink. Before your long run, stash water and a sports drink at 2.5-mile intervals. Fluids help flush waste products and deliver nutrients to repair muscle tissue.

Stretch. After a run, stretch your calves, hamstrings, and Achilles. Then do this hip stretch: Lie on your back and bend your right leg so your right ankle rests on your left knee. Pull your left knee toward you until you feel a stretch in your right buttock and hip. Hold for 10 to 15 seconds, then switch legs. Repeat three times.

Chill. Ease muscle soreness with a 20-minute soak in a tub of cold water, four trays of ice, a half cup of Moriah Dead Sea Salts, and a half cup of Origins Sensory Therapy Muscle Easing Bath Soak.

BY BRIAN METZLER

Blaze Any Trail

Seven all-terrain tips for your off-road steps

Pretend you're in a slasher flick, being chased through the woods by a chain saw–wielding madman. Twigs are snapping, and you're stumbling over rocks and ducking under tree limbs until, inevitably, you trip on a root. *Crack* goes your ankle, *whap* goes your body on the hard dirt. The madman catches up, the camera pans up to the full moon, and the screen fades to black.

That would never happen to Dave Mackey. As the 2003 US 50-mile trail-running champion and a four-time winner of the grueling Breckenridge Crest Trail Marathon in Colorado, Mackey runs on rocks like sprinters run on rubber tracks. He would have used short, compact strides to elude his pursuer. He would have spotted the root yards in advance. He would have ultimately left the freak doubled over and sucking wind.

If you want to run in the jungle, there's a steep price of admission, payable through either preparation or ER visits. That's why we chased Mackey through the woods near Boulder, Colorado, in search of seven ways to get dirt-worthy faster.

1. Don't Rush into Anything

Your first time on any trail is like your first time in the sack with a woman: It'll probably end sooner than you hoped. And if things go wrong, there might be first aid involved. That's okay, says Mackey. It takes time to get comfortable, to know when to accelerate and when to coast. On your virgin run, aim for 75 percent of your normal pace, paying attention to landmarks (sharp left after the walnut tree, watch out for jagged boulder). As you transition from the roads to dirt, you can work your way up to 100 percent effort; it takes time to learn the technical side of trail running. You'll be surprised at how much speed you can pick up once you know what's coming.

2. Keep Your Back Straight

Big hills leave even the best trail runners sucking wind. Your natural reaction is to hunch forward like Quasimodo, but that's a great way to keep your lungs from getting a full tank of gas. So do like Mackey and let your ankles adjust to the incline, keeping your back erect and using powerful, compact arm swings to propel yourself up the trail.

Essential Skill: Wiping Out

Falling properly can save more than just your wrists—it can also prevent your ankles from snapping or your back from being wrenched. When you feel yourself going down, scout out a soft zone and push in that direction. Like a stuntman, minimize the amount of surface area that hits the ground by tucking your chin and arms and landing on your side. To lessen the force of the impact, roll when you hit.

"I shorten my stride by a third or more but maintain the same cadence," says Mackey. Because you're moving more slowly, you won't need to look as far down the trail. But resist the temptation to watch your feet as you climb. Feet really aren't that interesting.

3. Snap a Mental Picture

You'll move faster down hills, so you need to be more aware of the terrain ahead. Mackey looks three or four paces beyond his feet, letting his brain place his footsteps based on that mental snapshot. Keep your weight back slightly—as if you're quick-stepping down the hill on your heels—and swing your arms with bent elbows up high, near your chest. Hold your arms out just far enough from your sides to ensure good balance. "Animals use their tails to shift weight," Mackey explains. "You're doing the same thing with your arms." On scree, or loose gravel, drop your arms to lower your center of gravity, and take shorter, gentler steps.

4. Stay Low

The taller your kicks, the harder you'll fall. So go with your favorite running shoes on anything but the nastiest turf. They're lower to the ground than are trail shoes, which have added cushioning that reduces stability and accentuates any rock-induced roll. The human body was designed to run off-road anyway, so unless your feet are particularly dainty, you'll be fine.

5. Take the High Road

Hill workouts are a great way to strengthen your legs, shorten your stride, and build up your stamina for longer runs. Try running hills that take at least 1 minute to ascend. If you're running intervals, shoot for 3- to 4-minute climbs; anything longer and you'll become too tired to get a quality workout.

6. Add Trail Mix to Your Training

Just like on-road prep, trail training requires a mix of short runs (between 20 minutes and an hour, two or more times a week) and LSD, or long, slow distance runs (an hour or so, once a week). But you'll also need to work in some hills and fartlek (Swedish for "speed play"—a random mix of easy runs and bursts of speed) to make it through a serious trail race, says Mackey. In one of Mackey's typical fartlek workouts, he alternates between moderate- and fast-paced spurts that last between 3 and 8 minutes.

7. Light Up

Once you've honed your trail intuition to spot obstacles on autopilot, hit the course at

When Animals Loiter Nearby

Man might rule the concrete jungle, but it's the forest folk you'll answer to once the pay phones start to thin.

"If you come across an animal, give it the right of way," says Douglas Inkley, senior science advisor at the National Wildlife Federation. Here's how to survive the most common close encounters of the toothy kind.

Skunk

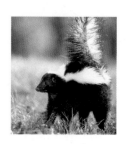

Where to watch out: Nationwide
What to do: Forget the stench— it's the rabies you should be worried about (although even that is quite rare). Melt into the background and disappear, particularly if the skunk seems agitated or is making strange noises. We're not sure what *normal* skunk noises are, but use your intuition.

Wild Boar

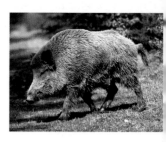

Where to watch out: California, North Carolina, Tennessee, West Virginia

night. It'll train you to respond to even fewer visual cues, making your running style more natural. A powerful but lightweight

What to do: They're short, stout, fast, and equipped with nasty tusks and nastier parasites. Climb a tree, hop on a rock, or just stand very still, and quietly slip away when you can, says Inkley. Boars have poor eyesight, so freezing in place might suffice.

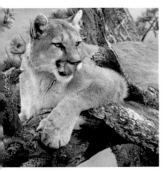

Mountain Lion

Where to watch out: Florida Everglades, Texas, western United States

What to do: Run away and you'll just attract attention, says Inkley. To avoid becoming kitty chow, yell, scream, make a commotion, and use threatening objects (sticks, stones, glossy photos of Clay Aiken) to get the lion to back off.

Grizzly Bear

Where to watch out: Alaska, northwestern United States

What to do: If you see a bear in the distance, make sure it stays there. If you're face-to-face with a growling grizzly (particularly one with cubs), just fall down and play dead. At medium distances, walk away calmly and deliberately, trying not to tremble in fear.

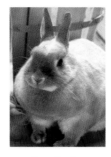

Copperhead

Where to watch out: From southwest Massachusetts west to Nebraska and south to the Florida panhandle; Texas

What to do: Back off immediately—freezing in place will only threaten the snake, says Inkley. If it strikes, immobilize the limb (don't try to suck out the poison, Rambo-style) and seek immediate help.

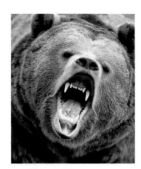

Rabbit

Where to watch out: Everywhere

What to do: Be vewwy, vewwy careful. The furball isn't likely to fly at your jugular, but don't get too close. Even the kinder, gentler denizens of the forest can carry rabies. Your best bet is to toss it a carrot and keep on trucking.

running headlamp (we like Black Diamond's 4.9-ounce Zenix, $45; bdel.com) should give you all the light you need. Headlamps also help you squeeze in after-work runs in the fall and winter.

BY TED SPIKER

Your Cross to Bear

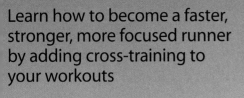

Learn how to become a faster, stronger, more focused runner by adding cross-training to your workouts

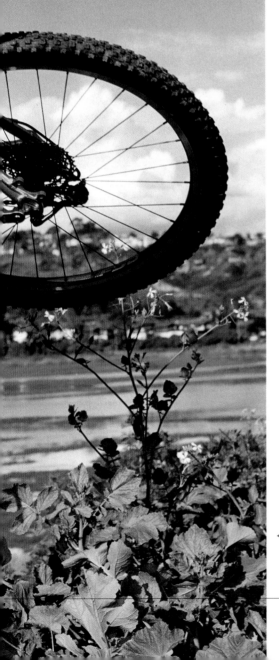

Runners need more than cramp-proof quads and lungs the size of hot-air balloons. To maximize performance and minimize injury risk, you should take a total-body approach—training your upper body as much as your lower body, your core as much as your limbs, and your brain as much as your heart.

"To be a strong, healthy runner, you need the whole package: endurance, speed, flexibility, coordination, and mental focus," says Neal Butler, CSCS, the track and cross-country coach at Grace College in Indiana. "You might be strong in one area, like endurance. But a weakness in another area, like flexibility, could prevent your ability from coming through." To develop and fine-tune your leg- and lung-powered engine, we asked athletes who rely on their shoulders, abs, and minds for their top workout methods and approaches. Add their expert advice to your routine, and you'll train smarter and run better.

Endurance
ROBYN BENINCASA, ADVENTURE RACER

What you can learn: For Robyn Benincasa, 26.2 miles is a sprint. Her races—which include everything from biking and running to climbing and paddling—typically last several days and hundreds of miles, so she needs the endurance to go as long as

◄ **ROBYN BENINCASA, Adventure Racer**
For Benincasa, building endurance is about challenging your mind and body. Ride a bike, go for a hike. Push yourself in new ways. (See page 162.)

she can as fast as she can. Endurance is everything for the distance runner, of course. While you might think your weekly long run has got you covered, Benincasa says there's another important component to endurance: the mental aspect. "Endurance is based on life experience," says Benincasa, 38, one of the sport's elite racers and captain of Team Merrell/Zanfel Adventure. "Whether you think something is long or not is completely dependent on what you've done before. You can boost your endurance by doing things that are mentally and physically challenging."

What you can do: Before a race, Benincasa follows a 2- to 3-month buildup period, incorporating hills, intervals, and increased distance. But once every 3 months (and no sooner than 6 weeks before a big event), she recommends doing something ridiculously long and hard—for you. And it doesn't have to be running. "Throw the watch away and go climb a mountain or do something long and hard just to do it," she says. Ride 100

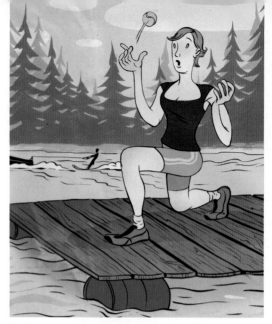

Challenge your core with juggling backward lunges.

miles on your bike or go on a day hike—anything, as long as it's considerably longer than your big race. It'll help you learn about such things as what to eat on long events and what anti-inflammatory medications work best, but it's a brain-builder more than anything. "It's more to get the mental edge," she says, "so that when you hit the wall, you have the confidence to keep going. You know you can break through and stick with it when it really sucks because you've done something that sucks worse."

Balance
KAREN TRUELOVE, WATER-SKIER

What you can learn: Waterskiing is a lot like running on a treadmill—with someone else randomly adjusting the speed. "Waterskiers are on a really unpredictable surface—it can be calm or almost oceanlike conditions," says Karen Truelove, 31, the 2002 USA Water Ski Female Athlete of the

PAINkiller

Shower Power
I've heard that taking a cold shower after a long run will lessen muscle soreness. Is this true?
K.I., Ithaca, New York

Yes, cold showers can cool down more than hormones. They can be helpful after hard workouts, when the muscles might have tiny tears and a buildup of waste products from vigorous exercise. Cold constricts the blood vessels in the muscles, and that reduces the amount of inflammation and soreness. It's like icing down a sore knee, only it's not as cold. This is the same treatment that champion racehorses receive. If it works for Triple Crown contenders, it's worth trying.

Year. With two forces—wind and water—constantly conspiring to throw Truelove off balance, she needs to train her body to stay balanced in unstable elements. But developing balance can also help runners—and not just trail runners and tipsy Hash House Harriers. With one foot off the ground at all times, runners are always somewhat off-balance. "Having balance is critical to injury-free running because it promotes stability and efficiency," says exercise physiologist Fred Schuster.

What you can do: Truelove does upper-body exercises, such as chest and overhead presses, on a stability ball instead of a bench. Steadying yourself on the ball works all the stabilizer muscles of your core that help keep you balanced. She also recommends the following exercises.

The partner ball toss: Stand on an unstable surface such as a foam roll or with one leg in the air. Have a partner toss a medicine ball to you. "Your partner shouldn't toss the ball straight at you," Truelove says. "The throw should be off center so you have to reach to catch it. That engages all kinds of muscle groups—your abs and your leg muscles are firing to keep you balanced."

Juggling backward lunges: Stand with your feet shoulder-width apart and a tennis ball or small medicine ball in one hand. Step back with your right foot in a backward lunge so your right knee almost touches the ground and your left thigh becomes parallel to the ground. As you're lunging, toss the tennis ball from one hand to the other. Alternate

legs, and repeat 16 to 20 steps. "It really challenges your balance when you have to do something with your upper body and lower body at the same time," Truelove says.

Power/Explosiveness
HOLLY MCPEAK, BEACH VOLLEYBALL PLAYER

What you can learn: In beach volleyball, everything is about power. "You need power

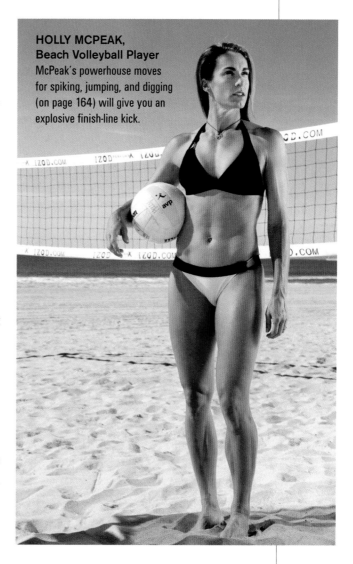

HOLLY MCPEAK,
Beach Volleyball Player
McPeak's powerhouse moves
for spiking, jumping, and digging
(on page 164) will give you an
explosive finish-line kick.

to jump, power to spike, power to leap to the side for a quick dig, and power to get into position in just one or two steps," says Holly McPeak, 35, a 2004 Olympic bronze medalist who has a record 72 beach titles. For McPeak, power is the difference between a win and a loss. For you, it's the difference between a personal record or a disappointment. "If your race comes down to the last 100 meters, that's where explosive training can pay off," Schuster says. "By training your fast-twitch muscles to fire very rapidly, you'll be able to generate more power to get across the finish faster."

What you can do: McPeak does a lot of core training to develop power. "That's where your explosive center is," she says.

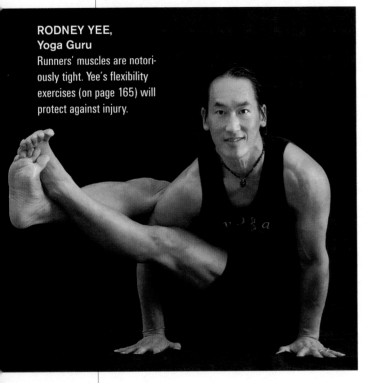

RODNEY YEE,
Yoga Guru
Runners' muscles are notoriously tight. Yee's flexibility exercises (on page 165) will protect against injury.

Here are three other moves from McPeak's training arsenal.

Explosive leg exercises: Instead of doing lower-body exercises like squats or lunges with heavy weights and slow, controlled movements, lower yourself slowly, and then jump up. Start with no weights or very light weights so you can focus on moving quickly.

Sprints: Ultrashort sprints train your body to accelerate into a finish-line kick. Mix sprints of 10 to 50 yards into your interval workouts.

Plyometrics: Plyometrics—jumping, bounding, hopping exercises—improve speed, strength, and joint stability, Schuster says. Hop onto a box or step with one or both feet, doing 15 to 20 repetitions at a quick pace. You can also vary it by jumping sideways or backward.

Flexibility
RODNEY YEE, YOGA GURU

What you can learn: While experts are busy debating the merits of stretching, runners often remain tighter than a pickle-jar lid. Our most inflexible areas tend to be the glutes, hamstrings, inner thighs, and hip flexors. That's because these muscles aren't able to stretch out naturally during the running motion, says the Yoda of yoga, Rodney Yee, 48, renowned instructor and author of *Moving toward Balance.* "Because running is a repetitive motion that uses the same muscles in the same way over and over, those muscles become increasingly tight," Yee says. Increasing your flexibility counteracts that tension, which improves your running stride and also protects against injury. When one muscle group is tight and an opposing group is flexible, it can lead to muscle imbalances and joint pain, Schuster says.

What you can do: Yee says there's no need to exert yourself by stretching too hard. "If you stretch too much, the muscles can rebel, causing damage," Yee says. Do these two yoga poses when your muscles are warm (after a run or a short warmup).

Cobbler's pose (inner thighs): Sit down on a yoga block or blanket with the soles of your feet pressed together. (Keep your back pressed against a wall for additional support.) Drop your knees so your inner thighs open up comfortably—don't push your knees all the way to the ground. Yee recommends putting yoga blocks or blankets under your knees. "When you give the body the message that it's being supported, your muscles let go even more," he says.

Downward dog (hamstrings and glutes): Place your hands and feet on the floor and, keeping your legs and arms straight, raise your butt up so that your body forms an inverted V. This stretches your hamstrings more efficiently than the ol' leg-on-fence stretch. "You do downward dog with an extended lower back instead of a rounded one, so the emphasis stays on the hamstrings," Yee says.

Upper-Body Strength
JOE JACOBI, WHITE WATER PADDLER

What you can learn: In white water slalom racing, Joe Jacobi competes not only against time and opponents but also against fiercely

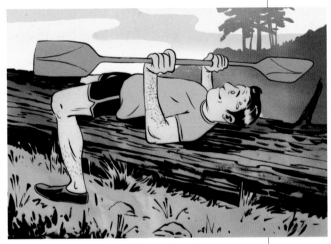
Upper-body strength improves your running form.

churning rapids. Jacobi, 35, a 1992 Olympic gold medalist, needs bull-like strength to fight currents and ballerina-like finesse to perform forward, backward, and steering strokes. Upper-body strength is also important to runners. It helps you maintain posture and endurance (if your upper body fatigues, your legs will soon follow, Butler says). Plus, a strong upper body generates more power and speed. "The rate of leg turnover is dictated to a large extent by arm motion," says Schuster.

What you can do: Strengthening the larger muscles in the upper body (chest, back, and shoulders) will help power your running. Jacobi's three-step routine hits these muscles.

The speed bench press (chest): Put about 50 percent of the weight of your maximum bench press on a barbell. Lying on a bench, lower the barbell about halfway down to your chest. Hold it for 3 or 4 seconds, then, in one quick movement, lift it to the top, lower it to your chest, then return it to the halfway point. Hold it again for 3 or 4 seconds, and repeat. Do two sets of 8 to 10 repetitions.

Pullups (back): "People tend to neglect their backs because they don't see them," Butler says. "But a strong back helps protect your form so you don't collapse forward when you're tired." If you can do two sets of eight pullups without cringing, add a dumbbell between your feet, like Jacobi does, to develop an even stronger back.

The empty can (shoulders): Jacobi does this exercise because it builds all the muscles—front, side, and rear—of his shoulders. Hold a light dumbbell (5 pounds or less) out in front of you with a straight arm at about 45 degrees from your body. Turn the dumbbell downward, like you're pouring a can of

soda. Lower your arm down to your thigh, then, keeping your hand turned, slowly raise your arm so your hand is at about eye level. Do two sets of 10 on each arm.

Time Management
SUSAN WILLIAMS, TRIATHLETE

What you can learn: By nature, triathletes seem to train more than they sleep—they have to log hours on the bike, in the pool, and on the road. Susan Williams, 35, the 2004 Olympic bronze medalist, once juggled three-a-day workouts, motherhood, and a part-time job with Lockheed Martin. Even if you're not training in three disciplines, you're no doubt tugged by work, family, and other responsibilities—and that's why time management is crucial for all runners. "You have to be able to set the other stuff aside and enjoy training," Butler says. "It's amazing to see how many people turn running—the stress reliever— into a stressor. If you're thinking about what you have to do while you're running, you might as well not be running."

What you can do: Williams says flexibility is key for fitting training into life. "I have a weekly plan, but it's not set in stone," she says. "You can see how you're feeling, what the weather conditions are like, and change things around a bit." Williams makes her training more manageable by organizing it into 2-week blocks instead of the standard training week. Being able to shuffle workouts within 14 days gives her more flexibility to schedule workouts around what else is happening in her life, business-wise, travel-wise,

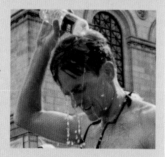

family-wise. And sometimes you've just got to suck it up and move your training to the back burner. "Athletes always struggle with taking time off," Williams says. "Remember that rest isn't only good for your body; it's also good to get caught up on other things you might have been missing while you were training. You'll appreciate your running more when you come back to it."

Mental Strength
PETER WHITTAKER, MOUNTAINEER

What you can learn: A 4- or 5-hour run might be tough, but try hiking to the top of Mount Rainier—a 30-hour event with only 4 or 5 hours of rest (granted, at a much slower, though still taxing, pace). Peter Whittaker, who's made more than 200 Rainier ascents as well as several expeditions on Everest, says climbing isn't necessarily about technical skill or physical conditioning. "I see more people fail on Mount Rainier not because they're physically unfit but because they couldn't go where they mentally needed to be," says Whittaker, 46, who co-owns Rainier Mountaineering guide services. "The people who perform best can deal with discomfort and the level of pain you experience when you're working at such extreme levels." Developing mental fortitude is useful during a race, but it also plays a role during training. "The key thing is that the mental is developed as much as the physical," Butler says. "You've got to be able to keep going and stay positive and pumped up. You have to persuade yourself to keep going all the time. If you're constantly

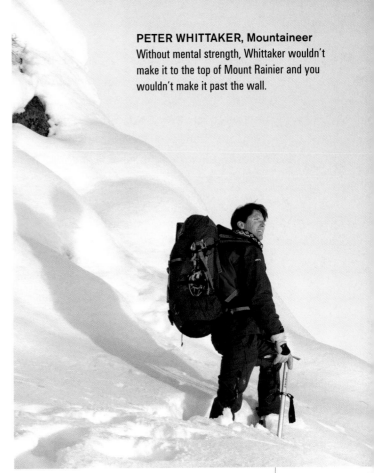

PETER WHITTAKER, Mountaineer
Without mental strength, Whittaker wouldn't make it to the top of Mount Rainier and you wouldn't make it past the wall.

talking yourself out of a workout, you're not going to go very far."

What you can do: When you're on a mountain, you can be hot, cold, hungry, thirsty, and just plain old uncomfortable. Much of the battle, Whittaker says, is that you have to be prepared to suffer. "My father once said that mountain climbing is like hitting yourself in the head with a hammer. It feels damn good when you stop." Whittaker says the only way to get into that mental zone is to stop thinking, stop looking at your watch, stop calculating, and stop listening too much to your body. Instead, take your mind to a nice place (wherever works for you, be it a beach or a buffet). "Some of my clients are so used to controlling things," he says. "They have no control up on the mountain and they freak. The less you think, the better you do. Our bodies are amazing, and they can be amazing for a really long time."

Agility
CATHERINE REDDICK, SOCCER PLAYER

What you can learn: During any game, Catherine Reddick runs several miles, going straight, back, side to side—all while trying to steal, block, and clear the ball. So she has to have fast legs—and quick feet. "As a defender, I have to keep my feet moving so I don't get beat," says Reddick, 23, who won an Olympic gold medal on the 2004 US women's team. While agility will help on a trail run (or when sidestepping potholes), it can also be a useful training tool for improving overall performance. "Doing agility drills and changing the way your body moves—zigzagging instead of going in a straight line—is very beneficial for runners," Schuster says. "These exercises build ankle and knee stability and teach your body how to change directions without losing speed, balance, or body control."

What you can do: Reddick does a lot of jumping and hopping drills, then goes directly to a sprint, to help train her feet to move quickly through uncertain terrain. This is her favorite exercise for faster feet and better balance.

The star drill: Set up five cones (or other markers) in a pattern like the points of a star, then place a sixth cone in the middle. Each cone should be about 8 to 10 feet from the center cone. Start at the center cone and sprint to one cone. Make a quick, tight circle around that cone and return to the center. Circle the center cone and continue to the

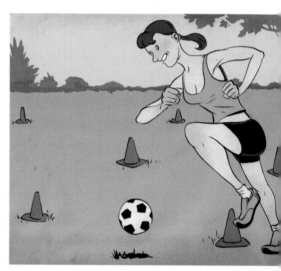

Agility drills improve balance and stability.

next cone in a clockwise direction, until you finish all points of the star. Rest for 30 seconds to 1 minute, and then repeat the sequence counterclockwise. "Keep working at it until you can go at top speed," Reddick says.

Core Strength
MARY SETTERHOLM, SURFER

What you can learn: To surf, it may seem like all you need is a board, some wax, and the ability to use "dude" as any part of speech. But even more important is having a strong core—your abdominals, lower back, and hips. "There's no solid ground when you're surfing and paddling, so your stability has to come from your core," says Mary Setterholm, 50, a former US surfing champion and director of the Surf Academy in California. "You need to move from your center because of the lack of stability. Your core is what grounds you." In running, core strength keeps your body aligned so it moves more efficiently. It's also crucial for absorbing shock. "When you hit the ground, the muscles in your trunk contract immediately to take the force of impact," Butler says. "A strong core is protective—it means you're hitting the ground; the ground isn't hitting you."

What you can do: Setterholm says the best core workout is paddling on a surfboard. Don't have a long board handy? Here are two core-building alternatives.

Paddling on a stability ball: Lie on a stability ball facedown, with your hips and stomach on the ball. Put your hands on the floor and raise your legs off the ground. Bend at the knee and alternate kicking mo-

tions with each leg. At the same time, raise one hand off the floor at a time and extend it out in front of you. The move simulates paddling, with your core trying to keep you balanced.

Curb jumps: Stand facing away from a curb with your heels about a foot from the curb. Jump back and land on the curb in a crouch with your knees bent. (Your feet should be slightly turned; picture yourself standing on a surfboard.) Jump back down. Jump up and down quickly all the way down a block. "This move takes a lot of concentration and really works your core," Setterholm says.

BY ADAM BEAN

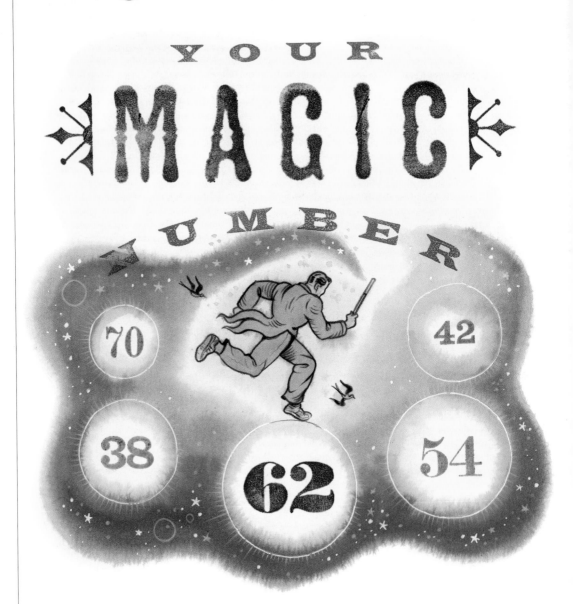

YOUR **MAGIC** NUMBER

For decades runners have been asking a simple question: How fast should my training runs be? Unfortunately, there hasn't been a simple answer. Until now

Unless you have a room at the Olympic Training Center in Colorado Springs, there's probably a lot of guesswork that goes into your training: How often to do hills? When to stretch, and for how long? What kind of recovery to take between hard runs?

Thanks to Jack Daniels, PhD, renowned coach and exercise physiologist, one thing that won't require guesswork anymore is your training speed. All you need to know is your VDOT number, a measurement Daniels came up with to reflect a runner's fitness level. Specifically, your VDOT is the amount of oxygen you consume during a minute of running. (VDOT is actually shorthand for "V-dot-O2 max," but don't worry, we won't go there.) This number, or value, can be determined in a research lab for a small fortune—or you can determine your VDOT from your recent race times. A 50-minute 10-K time, for example, corresponds to a VDOT number of 40.

The faster the race time, the higher the fitness level, the higher the VDOT. But here's the best part: You can use your VDOT to determine precisely how fast you should do your training runs. That's because at every level of fitness, according to Daniels, there are particular training speeds that provide optimal benefit. Daniels goes into detail on this in his new book, *Daniels' Running Formula*, but in "What's Your VDOT?" on page 172, we've made it easy for you by focusing on the three most important training speeds: easy pace, tempo pace, and interval pace. Once you find your VDOT number and optimal training paces, consult our 6-week VDOT-based 5-K training program so you can put theory into practice. It's the essence of customized training, and it works.

The Good Doctor

A true gentleman scholar, Jack Daniels medaled twice in the modern pentathlon at the 1956 and 1960 Olympics, studied sport in Sweden, once coached the Peruvian national distance team, and in 2000 was named NCAA Division III women's cross-country coach of the 20th century after a stellar career at SUNY-Cortland. He now coaches elite runners on the Nike Farm Team. Daniels, 71, lives in Cortland, New York, and has been contributing to *Runner's World* (which is published by the same company as *Men's Health*) for more than 2 decades.

A Perfect 5-K

Now it's time to try your own VDOT-based training program for a 5-K, the most popular race distance. VDOT training will likely be new for you, so it's best to start with a short race that will take only 6 weeks to train for. If it works, use your VDOT training paces when you train for longer distances as well. In your 5-K training, keep these things in mind:

Work up to it. You should be running at least 15 miles per week before starting this program. Total beginners should work up to this amount by running three or four times a week for 3 or 4 miles at a time, mixing in periodic walk breaks when needed.

Ease into speed. With Tuesday intervals, consider doing your first several repeats at slightly slower than VDOT-interval pace, then do your final one to two repeats at slightly faster than interval pace. This will

What's Your VDOT?

How to Use the Table

First, look for your most recent race time in one of the columns on the left, then move across to the middle to find your VDOT number. (If you've run more than one race distance lately and your corresponding VDOTs aren't the same, use the higher one.) Next, from your VDOT number, look across the table to find the training paces you should run for your easy, tempo, and interval workouts. Easy workouts will strengthen your running muscles. Tempo workouts will boost your lactate threshold, meaning you'll be able to run faster for longer. Interval sessions will increase your VO_2 max level, which will enable your body to process oxygen more efficiently. *Note:* Interval pace is given in per-400-meter pace below; 400 meters is roughly equivalent to a quarter-mile, or once around a standard running track.

5-K	10-K	HALF-MARATHON	MARATHON	VDOT	EASY PACE (PER MILE)	TEMPO PACE (PM)	INTERVAL PACE (400 M)
30:40	63:46	2:21:04	4:49:17	30	12:40	10:18	2:22
29:05	60:26	2:13:49	4:34:58	32	12:04	9:47	2:14
27:39	57:26	2:07:16	4:22:03	34	11:32	9:20	2:08
26:22	54:44	2:01:19	4:10:19	36	11:02	8:55	2:02
25:12	52:17	1:55:55	3:59:35	38	10:35	8:33	1:56
24:08	50:03	1:50:59	3:49:45	40	10:11	8:12	1:52
23:09	48:01	1:46:27	3:40:43	42	9:48	7:52	1:48
22:15	46:09	1:42:17	3:32:23	44	9:27	7:33	1:44
21:25	44:25	1:38:27	3:24:39	46	9:07	7:17	1:40
20:39	42:50	1:34:53	3:17:29	48	8:49	7:02	1:36
19:57	41:21	1:31:35	3:10:49	50	8:32	6:51	1:33
19:17	39:59	1:28:31	3:04:36	52	8:16	6:38	1:31
18:40	38:42	1:25:40	2:58:47	54	8:01	6:26	1:28
18:05	37:31	1:23:00	2:53:20	56	7:48	6:15	1:26
17:33	36:24	1:20:30	2:48:14	58	7:34	6:04	1:23
17:03	35:22	1:18:09	2:43:25	60	7:22	5:54	1:21
16:34	34:23	1:15:57	2:38:54	62	7:11	5:45	1:19
16:07	33:28	1:13:53	2:34:38	64	7:00	5:36	1:17
15:42	32:35	1:11:56	2:30:36	66	6:49	5:28	1:15
15:18	31:46	1:10:05	2:26:47	68	6:39	5:20	1:13
14:55	31:00	1:08:21	2:23:10	70	6:30	5:13	1:11

teach you to finish your runs and races strong.

Run comfortably hard. Thursday tempo workouts shouldn't leave you exhausted. The first half of the workout should feel very doable, even easy, with things only getting "interesting" at the end of the session.

Consider your options. Wednesdays are your "option" days. If you feel fine after Tuesday intervals, go 3 miles easy. If you feel fatigued or simply want to be sure you're ready and rested for tempo on Thursday, take Wednesday off.

Go long—but slow. Do your Sunday long runs at the same pace as your easy days. The point here is to build endurance, which will come in handy as you enter the third mile of your 5-K goal race.

Be wary. If you feel unusual fatigue for 2 or 3 consecutive days, take 2 rest days in a row and skip your next (planned) quality workout, whether that's an interval or tempo session. Same thing with pain. If something doesn't feel right and stays with you more than a day, shut it down for 2 days, and come back with a couple days of easy running.

Ease it back. Be diligent about your taper the week before your race. That means a couple of extra days of rest, dropping down to 200-meter repeats rather than 400 meters, and changing the Thursday tempo run to easy running and strides.

Race smart. On race day, follow the same routine as on your interval days. That is, jog easily for 10 minutes, stretch, and finish with four 100-meter pickups just before the start. When the gun sounds, you should be loose and your heart rate should be elevated. Run the first mile slightly slower than your goal pace, the middle mile at race pace, and the final mile a little faster than race pace.

WEEK	MONDAY	TUESDAY	WEDNESDAY	THURSDAY	FRIDAY	SATURDAY	SUNDAY
1	3 miles easy	4 × 400m interval pace	3 miles easy or rest	15 minutes tempo	Rest	4 miles easy	4 miles easy
2	3 miles easy	5 × 400m interval pace	3 miles easy or rest	20 minutes tempo	Rest	4 miles easy	4 miles easy
3	3 miles easy	6 × 400m interval pace	3 miles easy or rest	20 minutes tempo	Rest	4 miles easy	5 miles easy
4	3 miles easy	7 × 400m interval pace	3 miles easy or rest	25 minutes tempo	Rest	4 miles easy	6 miles easy
5	3 miles easy	8 × 400m interval pace	3 miles easy or rest	25 minutes tempo	Rest	4 miles easy	7 miles easy
6	Rest	8 × 200m interval pace	Rest	4 miles easy w/8 × 100m interval pace	3 miles easy	Rest	5-K race

Training Tips

I run 3 miles three to four times per week. Is that enough to stay fit?

D.K., HADLEY, MASSACHUSETTS

Your 3-miler every other day will certainly help maintain basic fitness, but you may want to consider adding some variety. Why? When you have a unique purpose for each run, you'll stay motivated. Don't panic—we're not talking about drastic changes. But on the weekend, for example, alternate between a slower and longer run one week, and a faster and shorter run or a 5-K race the next week. The longer run will build endurance and bring you a feeling of satisfaction. The shorter, faster run or race will boost your aerobic capacity.

One run a week can be your "fast" day. Just a few 90-second accelerations during an otherwise easy run will improve muscle performance. And 1 day per week should be fun. Many runners experience burnout because they don't regularly schedule social runs or try a route through new and interesting areas. Variety is the spice of running— and it doesn't take much of a change to make any run more interesting.

ON THE SURFACE

Is it better to run on a treadmill or outside?

J.R., BOISE, IDAHO

The workout is about the same, but some experts advise setting a treadmill's incline at 1 percent to mimic the effort needed on roads. Most doctors will tell you a treadmill is better because it's easier on the knees. But if running indoors is so unappealing that you skip workouts, go outside—just choose your surface carefully. Concrete is the

TOP SPEED

Call Up Your Reserves

Research shows your body maintains a reserve during exercise. In a study published in *Medicine and Science in Sports and Exercise*, researchers used a slowed-down clock to trick men into thinking they were pedaling at top effort for 30 seconds, when it was actually 36 seconds. Their power output dropped sharply in the final 3 seconds. "The brain can be deceived to within 10 percent of the actual distance or time," says study author Les Ansley, PhD. To tap into your reserve, Ansley suggests training at your 10-K pace for a slightly longer distance than 10 kilometers so you learn to maintain a fast pace longer.

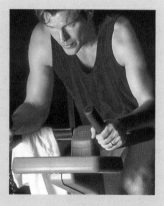

worst, with asphalt close behind. Grass or a dirt path is best. Stick to an even surface and replace your shoes every 6 months or 300 to 500 miles.

FUEL UP

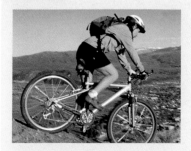

Get Your Carb Boost

Don't sweat the types of carbohydrates you consume on a long bike ride or run. A study in the *Journal of Strength and Conditioning Research* shows that you'll get an equal boost from foods whether they have a low glycemic load (like apples) or a high one (like crackers). Lead study author Conrad Earnest, PhD, says that drinking only water is sufficient for sessions under 90 minutes, but for longer periods, you should consume 25 to 40 grams of carbohydrates every 30 minutes to fuel your body.

CHUG IT DOWN

Do sports drinks really hydrate you faster than plain old, calorie-free water?
T.U., SPRINGFIELD, NEW HAMPSHIRE

The $1.50 you pay for Gatorade is worth it, according to Leslie Bonci, MPH, RD, director of sports nutrition at the University of Pittsburgh Medical Center. A good sports drink contains carbohydrates as well as sodium, which together expedite the movement of fluid out of the belly and into your muscles. Water also tends to satisfy thirst earlier in the process than it should, which is problematic because you might not take in

enough fluid, says Bonci. Yet the opposite can also be true with water. "There seems to be a limit to how much sports drink a person will consume," says Bonci, but it is possible to drink more water than a body needs. The flavors and price are two reasons Gatorade overload isn't seen much. The perfect amount? Per hour of exercise, a minimum of 20 ounces, maximum of 40 (one to two bottles). If you sweat heavily or are exercising in hot weather, err toward two bottles. For the fastest hydration, look on the nutrition labels for drinks with 100 milligrams of sodium per 8 ounces.

MUSCLE UP

Going Downhill Fast

In a recent study published in the *Journal of Applied Physiology,* scientists found that running downhill helps a rat develop its all-important spinotrapezius—a muscle with a fiber composition similar to that of the human quadriceps. For us, running on any decline stresses the quadriceps and gluteals, says study

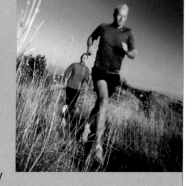

author David Poole, PhD. Running downhill puts these muscles under "almost three times as much force as level or uphill running" and builds the quads, Poole says.

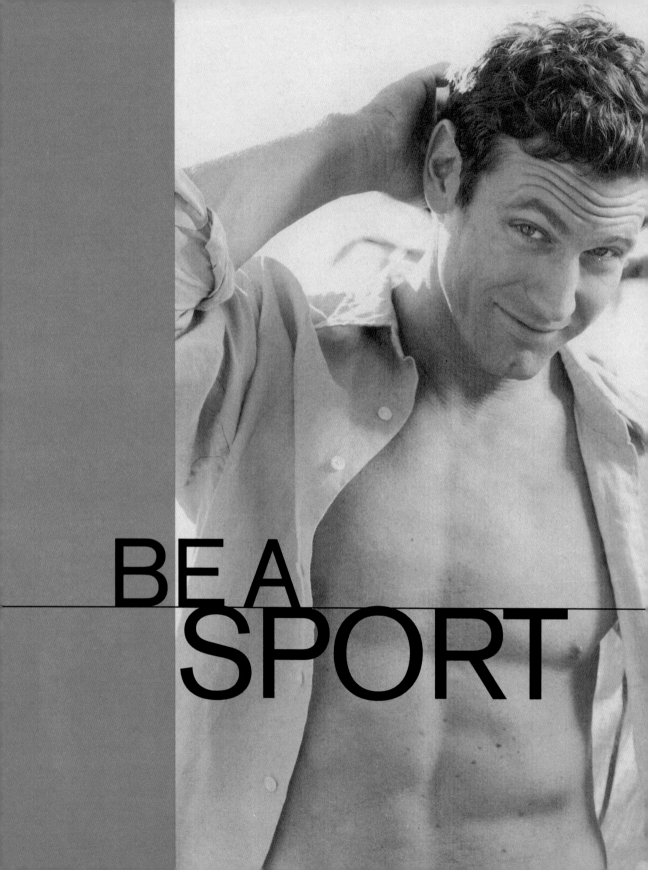

BE A
SPORT

As kids if we couldn't throw, hit, kick, ride, or paddle something, we weren't interested.

Some things don't change.

We still live to play and play to win. And win you will. No matter what your sport, this is the ultimate guide to beating the other guy. With the masterful moves in this section, you'll run faster, swing harder, hit farther, jump higher, and serve stronger than ever before. Plus you'll strengthen the typical trouble spots for your sport, so you can play without pain. Or satisfy the thrill-seeker in you and take on a new challenge—like catching big air off of a mountain. Everything you need before you take off is in these pages. Except the guts. Do *you* have it in you?

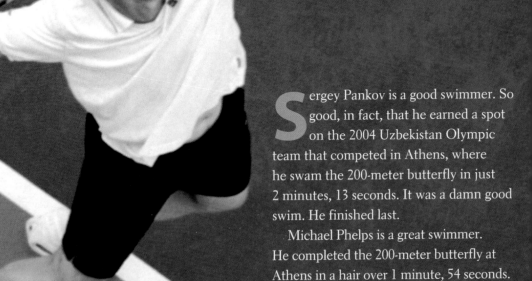

BY TREVOR THIEME

Raise Your Game

If you want to play with the big boys, you've got to train like them. Here's how to be on the top of your game, no matter what your sport

Sergey Pankov is a good swimmer. So good, in fact, that he earned a spot on the 2004 Uzbekistan Olympic team that competed in Athens, where he swam the 200-meter butterfly in just 2 minutes, 13 seconds. It was a damn good swim. He finished last.

Michael Phelps is a great swimmer. He completed the 200-meter butterfly at Athens in a hair over 1 minute, 54 seconds. It was a damn great swim. He won the gold.

You're probably more like Pankov—good at a handful of sports but truly great at very few, maybe none. That's because being good requires only natural ability. Being great, however, demands that you nurture your genetic advantage with hard work, disciplined training, and a commitment to constant improvement—on and off the court (or field or trail).

If you want to take your game to the next level, consider this your playbook. First we tackle the seven burning questions in sports fitness. For answers, we picked the brain of Mark Verstegen, MS, CSCS, a trainer who's worked with pro athletes in every sport. He's also president of Athletes' Performance in Tempe, Arizona, and author of *Core Performance* (Rodale 2004). Incorporate his tips into your daily routine—shoot for three sets of 5 to 10 reps—and you'll be swinging harder, running faster, and jumping higher in no time.

We also target the 10 most difficult sport-specific moves, from reading a golf green to throwing a knuckleball. Then, with the help of a team of experts, we dissect them and explain how you can immediately make them part of your game. So read, heed, and become unbeatable in your sport.

How can I run faster?

There are many aspects to running fast—cruising speed, breakaway speed—but the most important is acceleration. "It makes up 85 to 90 percent of the movement in sport," Verstegen says, "especially if you play on a team." Take soccer: Having a fast 40-meter sprint time won't necessarily help you beat your opponent to the ball, but

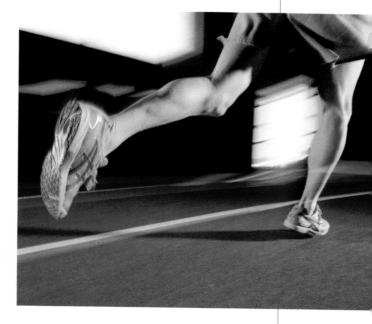

being able to outaccelerate him during the first 10 to 20 meters will. Same with basketball: First-step quickness will determine whether your fast break ends in a basket or a block.

Many coaches and athletes believe that speed is genetic, and that no matter how hard you train, you simply can't improve on natural ability. While it's true that some athletes will always exhibit greater talent, you can enhance your acceleration by increasing your stride length and frequency. Stride length is dictated by your range of motion and the power you release into the ground with each step. Stride frequency is determined by technique, biomechanics, and the performance of your fast-twitch muscle fibers (as opposed to slow-twitch fibers, which, when well conditioned, give you great endurance). Here are a few exercises to get you started.

FORWARD LUNGE/FOREARM TO INSTEP

Although this exercise improves flexibility in the legs, torso, and back, its most important benefit is increasing hip separation—a critical component of stride length. Step forward with your left leg as if doing a lunge (A), and then place your right hand on the ground so it's even with your left foot and supporting your weight. Then take your left elbow and reach down to the instep of your forward leg while keeping your back knee off the ground (B). Move your left hand outside your left foot and push your hips toward the sky (C). Finally, step forward into your next lunge (D) and repeat.

A
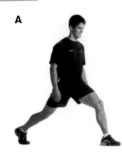

B
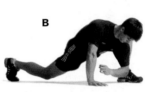

C
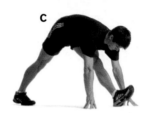

D
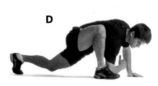

GET-UPS

These will help you develop proper acceleration biomechanics. Start by getting into a pushup position—feet together—then bring your left foot forward, stand up, and explode into a sprint

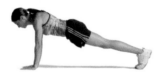

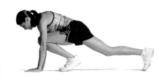

with pistonlike leg and arm action. Run 10 yards, stop, and repeat.

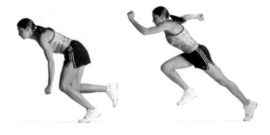

SPLIT JUMPS

Next, you'll need horsepower. Take a large step forward, keeping your chest up, shoulders back, and knees and toes straight. Move your hips back and down until your back knee nearly touches the ground. Hold this position for 2 seconds, then explode up with your hips and legs while throwing your arms up. Extend your front leg and land in the original split-squat position. Repeat several times and switch legs.

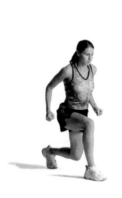
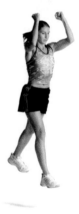

How can I swing harder?

A common misconception about swinging harder is that it depends on arm strength. The truth is, you can have the strongest arms in the world and still struggle to hit the ball to the outfield. If you want a stronger swing—regardless of whether you're holding a bat, club, racket, or fist—you've got to focus on your hips, torso, and shoulders (i.e., your pillar). "You'll have to be able to transfer power efficiently from your feet, through your hips, into your shoulders, and out into your arms and hands," Verstegen says. "That's what allows people to take a 20-yard jump in their drive, achieve monstrous spikes, and hit baseballs out of the park." To achieve a powerful swing, mix the following exercises into your weekly routine.

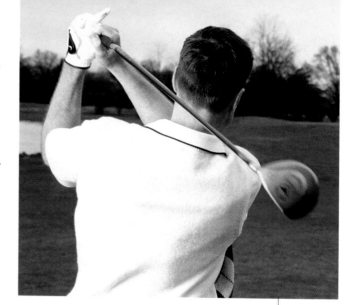

PEAK
performance

Stronger Swing

Two studies on baseball players show that adding medicine-ball exercises to a strength-training program can help generate more bat speed. The moves condition the hips and torso, which can help you rotate faster. So whether your game is baseball, golf, or tennis, ignite your turning power with the medicine-ball routine here, which was presented at the 2004 annual meeting of the American College of Sports Medicine. Do two sets of six repetitions (on each side) of each exercise twice a week, suggests David Szymanski, PhD, CSCS, the lead study author. Every 4 weeks, use a slightly lighter ball and do two more reps per exercise.

THE MOVE	THE METHOD
HITTER'S THROW	Stand holding a medicine ball above your right shoulder. Then, as if you were swinging a baseball bat, straighten your arms across your body as you throw the ball as far as you can.
STANDING FIGURE-8	Pair up with a workout partner, stand with your backs to each other about 2 feet apart, and hold a medicine ball at midabdominal height. Rotate your torso quickly from right to left to hand the ball to your partner, who also rotates to receive the ball. Then rotate in the opposite direction to receive the ball on your right side.
SPEED ROTATION	Stand with your back to a partner (who stands a few feet away from you), both arms extended to your right at shoulder height. Your hands should face behind you. Now look over your right shoulder and have your partner toss the ball to your outstretched hands. Then rotate your torso as fast as you can, while swinging your straight arms to throw the ball back to him.
STANDING SIDE THROW	Same as the hitter's throw, but hold the ball at your hip instead of above your shoulder.

HIP CROSSOVERS

This will build mobility and strength into your torso by conditioning your hips to work independently of your shoulders. Lie faceup on the floor, and extend your arms and shoulders out to your sides while keeping your knees bent and feet flat on the ground. Twist your bent legs to the right until they reach the floor, then twist to the left. Once comfortable with this version, try it with your hips and knees bent 90 degrees, feet off the ground. For an added challenge, straighten your legs.

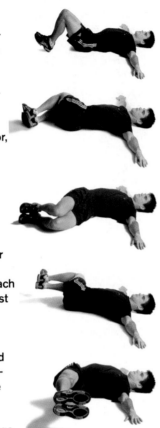

ONE-ARM ROTATIONAL ROW

This exercise will improve stability and strength in your back, torso, shoulders, and arms. Attach a handle to a low pulley on a cable machine and kneel perpendicular to it, keeping your right knee and left foot on the floor. Reach across your body with your right hand and grab the handle, turning your hips and shoulders to the machine. Now rotate your right shoulder back and pull the handle to your right hip. Do 10 reps, and repeat with your opposite side.

How do I develop breakaway speed?

"Breakaway speed is kind of like fifth gear," Verstegen says. "You're already cruising, and you just take off." It's what allows a wide receiver to pull away from a defensive back, an 800-meter runner to kick past his opponents, and a midfielder to gun it toward the opposing goal.

To acquire breakaway speed, you'll have to develop a fluid cyclical stride (as opposed to the pistonlike leg action of acceleration) and tremendous pillar strength. The latter is important because a stable pillar—hips, torso, and shoulders—is what allows you to transfer energy efficiently through your body.

Take sprinter Tim Montgomery: As he sprints, his torso hardly moves. Without that solid pillar, his movements would become sloppy, energy would "leak," and he'd never be able to cover 100 meters in 9.78 seconds (the world record). And he'd leave himself open to injury. Try these exercises.

PEAK
performance

Go for a Long Drive

Researchers have found that a free-weight program combined with plyometrics boosts golfers' driving distance. Six men on an 8-week program of weights and plyometric medicine-ball exercises (releasing the ball at the end of the move) improved their drives by 10 yards more than did five men who did aerobics and light machine weight training. The study in the *Journal of Strength and Conditioning Research* concludes that releasing the medicine ball trains the muscles to accelerate the swing through the ball. Start a total-body strength routine, and twice a week do three sets of eight simulated golf swings with a medicine ball, throwing it against a wall.

BACKWARD LUNGE WITH A TWIST

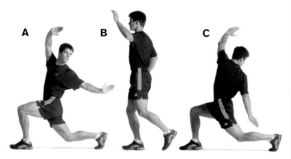

A   B   C

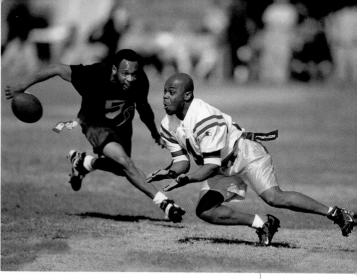

This will help free up your hips, which are critical for shifting into breakaway speed. With your feet together, step backward into a lunge with your right leg. Arch your back slightly while twisting your torso over your left leg, and reach your right hand toward the sky (A). Push out of that position and step back into your next lunge (B), this time with your left leg, twisting your torso to your right and reaching toward the sky with your left hand (C).

IN AND OUTS

This drill conditions your body for speed changes. Space five cones 20 yards apart on a field. Build up speed for the first 20 yards, put it into fifth gear for the second 20, take it down a notch and coast for 20 yards when you pass the third cone, then go all out again for the final 20 yards.

TUCK JUMPS

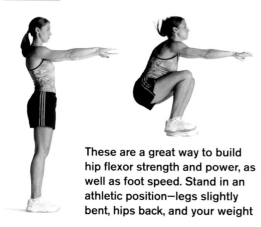

These are a great way to build hip flexor strength and power, as well as foot speed. Stand in an athletic position—legs slightly bent, hips back, and your weight on the middle to front part of your feet, arms in front—and explode off the ground, tucking your knees in front of your body as you jump. Land and repeat.

PILLAR BRIDGE

This exercise is great for developing pillar strength and total-body stability. Lie facedown in a prone pushup position, your forearms resting on the floor. Your elbows should be under your shoulders and bent 90 degrees. Push off your elbows, tuck your chin so your head is in line with your body, and pull your toes toward your shins. Change it up by lifting one arm or leg and holding it for 2 seconds, or lifting an opposite leg and arm, holding, and switching sides.

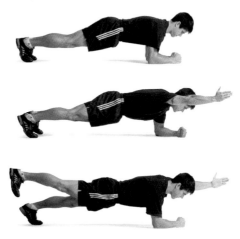

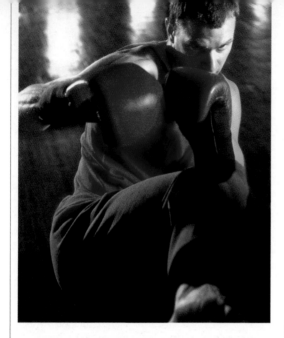

How can I sharpen my reaction time?

When a major league pitcher throws a fastball at 95 mph, it takes 0.39 seconds for it to cross home plate. Since the average player takes two-tenths of a second to swing a bat, he has 0.19 seconds to make the decision of whether to swing.

Think of reaction time as a processing loop. When a stimulus comes in—a visual or audible cue—it is interpreted by the brain, which then scans its library of archived actions for the most appropriate response. Once that response is selected, your brain instructs your muscles to contract and extend in the corresponding motor pattern. The more often you receive that stimulus, the more efficiently you'll process it, and the faster you'll react. "It's like a wagon trail becoming a superhighway," Verstegen says.

The best way to improve reaction time is with sport-specific activities, such as rapid-fire volleys and serve returns for tennis players, starting drills for swimmers and

sprinters, and drop-and-stand drills for football linemen. But you can also develop general reactive quickness by performing the following drills.

RAPID-RESPONSE DRILLS

Grab a partner and stand in position with your feet outside your hips. When your partner gives you an auditory cue—a clap, for example—start jumping from side to side as quickly as possible over an imaginary line. When your partner claps again, freeze. This exercise will sharpen your reaction time and quicken your nervous system's response time.

TURN AND CATCH

Assume a ready position, and have a partner stand several paces behind you with a tennis ball. Your partner will then toss the ball toward you and shout "Ball!" sometime after it leaves his hand. It's your job to turn around, locate the ball in midair, and catch it. To make this exercise more difficult, have your partner vary where he throws the ball—toward your head, shoulders, stomach, legs—and when he gives the cue.

HAND SLAP

You're probably familiar with this exercise from grade school. Have a partner stand in front of you with his hands held out, palms facing up. Place your hands on his, palms down, and try to pull your hands away when he flips his around to slap the backs of yours.

How can I become more agile?

Agility can be defined as multidirectional speed—the ability to rapidly change directions in up to 360 degrees of motion. Whether you're a soccer midfielder, a football quarterback, or a basketball forward, at some point you're going to have to stop, change direction, and accelerate again, all in a fraction of a second. And since this will happen in response to a stimulus—a pass or a rebound, for example—your agility goes hand in hand with reaction time (see previous question).

To improve your agility, you'll have to focus on three main areas: mobility (especially in your hips), dynamic balance, and elasticity, which you can think of as "springiness." The exercises that follow should do the trick.

LATERAL LUNGE

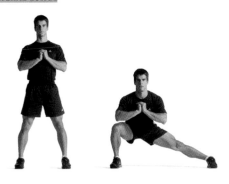

This will help improve flexibility in your hips and groin. Begin by standing in an athletic position and stepping out to the right, keeping your toes pointed straight and your feet flat. Squat down on your right leg, keeping your left leg straight and your weight on your right heel to midfoot.

Hold for 2 seconds, return to the standing position, and repeat.

LATERAL BOUND

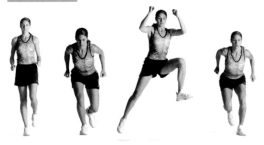

This will help you develop explosive cutting ability. Start by balancing on your right leg, then jump laterally and land on your left leg (be sure to have only one foot on the ground at a time). Hold for 3 seconds, and repeat to the other side.

THREE-HURDLE DRILL

This will help you develop lightning-quick feet and solid balance. Lay three obstacles on the ground (towels, books, cups), spaced 2 to 3 feet apart. Begin by straddling the first obstacle, then run laterally over the obstacles, never letting your feet cross. Rapidly reverse direction and repeat.

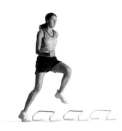

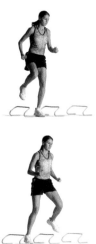

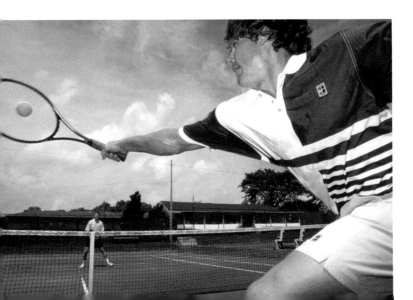

DROP LUNGE

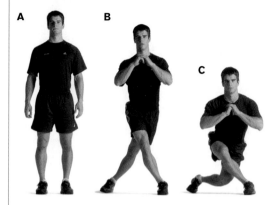

This exercise focuses on hip-and-glute flexibility. From your starting position (A), step back with your left foot until it's 2 feet to the outside of your right foot (B). Square your shoulders and feet. You want your chest up and tummy tight, and the majority of your weight on your right leg. Drop into a full squat by pushing your hips back and down while keeping your right heel on the ground (C). Now stand back up, driving hard with your right leg. Repeat for several steps to the right with the same leg, and then switch legs and move to your left.

How do I improve my vertical leap?

Verstegen gets this question more than any other. Vertical leap is measured by subtracting your standing reach from your jump reach; it's between 28 and 34 inches for most NBA players. To improve your vertical leap, you'll have to increase your relative strength, or the power you're able to produce pound for pound. You'll also need to develop the timing and coordination to fire all of your jumping muscles simultaneously.

Roughly 10 percent of your power will come from your calves, a third from your quads, another third from your glutes and hamstrings, and the rest from your back and

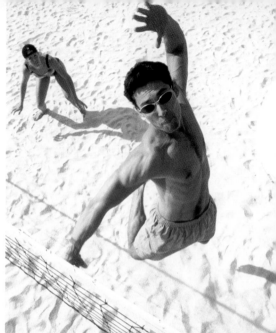

rector muscles. "Bringing all that power together is called a summation of forces," Verstegen says. "It's like when you snap a towel and all the energy is concentrated in a single pop!" Here's how to pop over defenders.

SQUAT JUMP

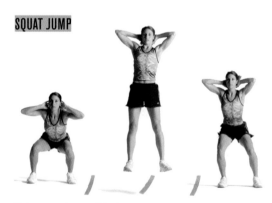

This exercise will help you build explosive power in your hips and legs. Stand in an athletic position with your feet outside your hips and your hands on your head. Keeping your back erect and your stomach tight, lower your hips until your thighs are parallel to the ground. Then jump, pushing up with your glutes and quads. Extend your ankles, knees, and hips in a straight line and land back in an athletic position.

SQUAT TO PRESS

This will help you develop total-body strength. Stand with dumbbells at shoulder height, elbows resting on your ribs, palms facing each other. Squat until the tops of your thighs are parallel to the floor, then explode up with your hips and quads, using the momentum to drive the weights over your head. Finish with your arms and legs straight. Lower the dumbbells to your shoulders, drop into a full squat, and repeat.

ROMANIAN DEADLIFT

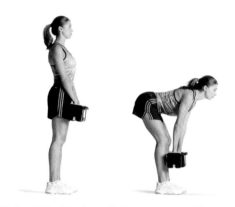

This will build strength in your hamstrings, glutes, and back. Grab a barbell with an overhand grip just wider than your shoulders, or stand holding a pair of dumbbells at your sides. Shift your hips back and lower the bar as far as you can while keeping your back straight. Don't think of the exercise as bending forward; think of it as sitting back, but with your torso moving forward instead of staying upright. Fire your hamstrings and glutes as you return to an upright position.

How can I improve my endurance?

To improve endurance, you have to understand how your body produces energy. During aerobic exercise, your body burns oxygen. But when you kick it into overdrive, there isn't enough oxygen to go around, so your body switches over to anaerobic metabolism, which produces energy in the absence of oxygen. The by-product is lactic acid, and the more it accumulates in your muscles, the more they'll ache and the less efficiently they'll work.

To improve endurance, therefore, you'll have to increase your lactic threshold—the point at which lactic acid begins to build up in your muscles—and the best way to do that is with interval training. "Intervals are to endurance what weight lifting is to strength," says Paul Robbins, the metabolic specialist at Athletes' Performance. "You overload the body to bring it to a higher level."

Plan your interval workout as part of a 3-day-a-week routine. On the first day, you'll perform low-intensity exercise that raises

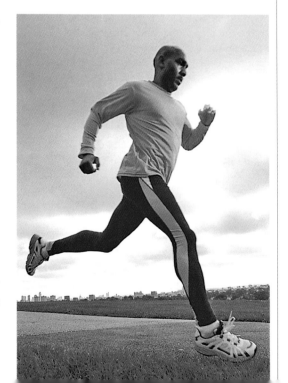

your heart rate to 65 percent of its maximum; this can be done by going for a light jog or bike ride. On the second day, you'll kick it up a notch by operating at 80 to 85 percent of your maximum heart rate. You can perform the same exercises you did on Day 1, as long as you raise your heart rate into the next zone. The third day is for intervals, where you'll elevate your heart rate to 90 percent of its maximum. Robbins recommends three 5-minute intervals, progressing as follows.

FIRST PROGRESSION

Spend the first minute at 80 to 85 percent of your max heart rate (let's call it Zone A), kick it up to 90 percent for a minute (Zone B), then spend the remaining 3 minutes back at 80 to 85 percent. A rule of thumb is to spend as much time recovering as you do exerting yourself, so follow your interval with 5 minutes of light exercise. Then move to the second progression.

SECOND PROGRESSION

Here, you'll alternate between Zones A and B in 1-minute intervals. Go all out for the first minute, taper back the second, go all out for the third, taper back on the fourth, and finish strong in Zone B. Exercise lightly for 5 minutes.

THIRD PROGRESSION

Finally, spend 2 minutes going as hard as you can in Zone B, taper back for a minute in Zone A, and then jump back into the top zone for the final 2 minutes.

The 10 Most Difficult Sport Moves . . . Made Simple

ROAD BIKING

How to Power Up a Steep Hill

Forget pumping the pedals. If you want to cycle faster and farther with less effort, you need to pedal in circles. Bill Strickland, executive editor of *Bicycling* magazine, offers instructions.

1. Throw down. Push down hard from the top of the stroke until the crankarms are horizontal.

2. Shuffle sideways. Pretend you're scraping mud off the bottom of your shoes from this point until the next time the crank arms are horizontal, and continue to exert force by pulling across the bottom of the stroke.

3. Pull up. Finish by pulling the pedal to the top of the stroke. Naturally, you'll need toe straps or a clipless pedal system to anchor your feet.

GOLF

How to Read a Green

The quickest way to shave strokes from your score is to turn three-putts into two-putts. Veteran golf pro Loren Roberts, aka "The Boss of the Moss" because of his uncanny ability to examine a green and grasp its nuances, explains how.

1. Harvest the grain. Grass rarely grows vertically. If there's a slope, gravity bends the blades down along it. If there's a nearby water source, the blades naturally grow to-

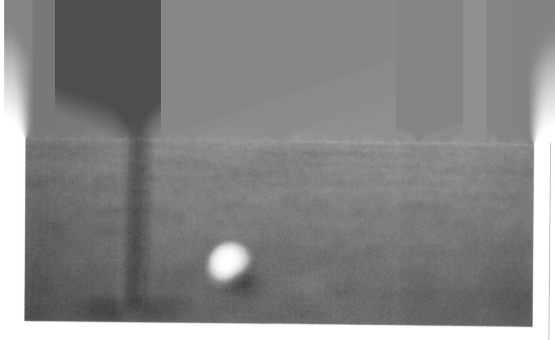

ward it. As the sun moves across the sky, the blades follow. Weigh all these factors and try to identify a general growing pattern, or "grain." Expect any putt along the grain to roll faster, and any putt against the grain to roll slower.

2. Gauge the slope. First, walk around on the green to get a general idea of its pitch. "It's a combination of what you feel with your feet and what you see with your eyes," says the Moss Boss. Then crouch behind your ball to determine if there's a tilt. If there is, walk to the downhill side and study the putt from there. It'll give you a surprisingly better perspective.

3. Picture pouring water. If you're still perplexed, imagine what would happen if you slowly poured water on the green. Hit your putt to follow the flow.

4. Don't aim. Next, just step up and hit the ball. "The more you aim and try to drop it in the center of the hole, the harder it is to

do," Roberts says. "Having good speed and the right distance is more important than getting the perfect line."

5. Use the practice green. If you have only a few minutes to warm up before your tee time, spend it practicing your putting.

PAINkiller

Par for the Course?
Most golfers I know get lower-back pain. For me, it's my upper back, right between my shoulder blades. Why?

C.O., Myrtle Beach, South Carolina

Golf can be a strain. The constant reaching, twisting, and swinging wreak havoc on your back muscles. That's why it's important to stretch for at least 15 minutes before playing—and keep it up during your round, between shots, to stay loose. In the gym, build up your back and shoulder muscles by performing reverse flies. Stand with your knees and elbows slightly bent, and hold a pair of light dumbbells with your palms facing each other. Bend forward at the waist until your back is almost parallel to the floor, then raise your arms straight out to the sides, maintaining the slight bend in your elbows. Pause when your arms are parallel to the floor, lower the weights, and repeat. The downside: You'll have no more excuses for a bad swing.

It'll help you gauge green speed and save you strokes later.

6. Putter around at home. Skip the swing set and get a backyard putting green instead. A 15-by-30-foot, four-hole model from Putting Greens International costs $7,000 (putting.com).

DOWNHILL SKIING

How to Turn a Mogul into a Molehill

Think of these snow-clad speed bumps as hurdles on a running track: They're meant to trip losers. Dan Egan, an extreme skier and author of *All-Terrain Skiing*, explains how to smooth them out. It requires practice, so take your first 50 at quarter-speed before trying to impress the snow bunnies.

1. Slow down. As soon as you see the first mogul, put your hands in front of your body and make a few gentle turns. Keep your head up and stay centered over your skis.

2. Hit it. About 15 feet before the mogul, relax your knees to brace for impact, keeping your torso straight. Bad skiers tend to bring their skis together; try to keep yours shoulder-width apart. As you climb the mogul, bend your knees.

3. Plant your pole. When you near the mogul's peak, reach out and plant a pole on its front, downhill slope. Use that as a turning point. Push on the pole with a fast snap of the wrist to turn atop the crest of the mogul.

4. Don't launch. As you pass the mogul's summit, put your entire weight on your toes and use the edges of your skis to control your speed. This will prevent you from catching air.

5. Recover and watch out. As you ski into the trough, straighten your knees. Be ready to do this again in a few seconds.

SNOWBOARDING

How to Catch Big Air

Seems like everybody and his mother fancy themselves snowboarders these days. The only way to rise above the rest is to rise above the rest . . . literally. Here's how to perform a jump with a minimum of trauma, according to Brian Delaney, co-owner of Delaney Adult Snowboard Camps in Aspen, Buttermilk, Beaver Creek, and Vail, Colorado.

1. Pick a line. Look for a jump with a smooth approach and an even smoother

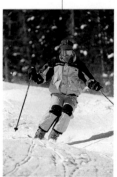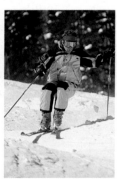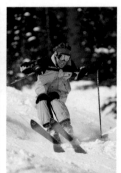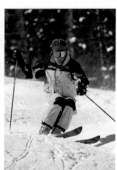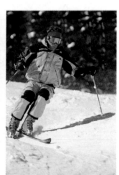

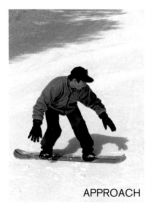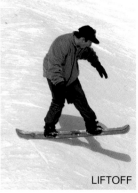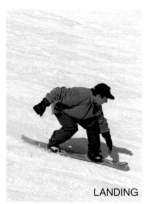

APPROACH   LIFTOFF   LANDING

landing spot. Adopt the ready position of a tennis player awaiting a hard serve, and loosen up. Start your glide. As you near the ramp, lower your body into the position shown.

2. Don't look up. Keep your board flat, your torso steady, and your eyes level. If your eyes go up, your head and body will follow (next stop: your ass). Launch yourself by firing your thigh muscles and blasting out the flex in your knees and ankles. Don't move anything else. Suddenly, you're flying! You've got about a second of airtime (Delaney can catch 4), so make the most of it. Hoot and holler, but keep your upper body in the position shown to ensure a stable flight.

3. Prepare for touchdown. As you approach Mother Earth, extend your landing gear in anticipation of impact. Act like a spring and absorb the mountain with your ankles and knees. Your weight should be evenly distributed over both legs and across the board. Touch down with the board parallel to the angle of the slope so the entire base meets snow. Now hit the brakes, turn around, and encourage your mom. She needs your help.

BASKETBALL

How to Make a Hook Shot

On the basketball court, a short guy can play taller—as long as he masters the hook shot. Pete Newell, a former Olympic basketball coach, explains the four-step sequence for nailing a hook shot. (If you're left-handed, reverse the instructions.)

1. Get set. With your back about 6 feet from the basket, stand at the right side of the lane. Bend your knees and hold the ball at chest height, elbows out.

2. Pivot. Turn your body quickly to the left and lift your right foot, keeping your left foot planted firmly. Keep the ball on the right side of your chest. Start looking for the rim.

3. Jump. When you can see the basket over your left shoulder, jump off your left foot. Raise the ball high in your right hand while you drop your left arm for balance. Even a taller defender will find it difficult to block the ball because you're shielding it with your body.

4. Release. Stiffen your right arm and wrist, and flick the ball toward the basket

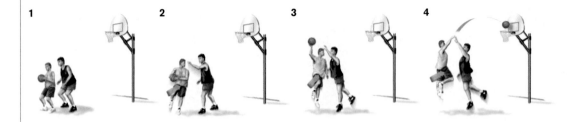

1 2 3 4

with your fingers. Aim for the square on the backboard; bank shots are more likely to go in than straight-on shots. You should land facing the basket so you have a fighting shot at a rebound—just in case.

TENNIS

How to Smash a Backhand

Do your tennis opponents torture you by playing to your soft-as-a-baby's-behind back-hand? We would, too. Here's a smashing one-handed response, courtesy of Dick Gould, head coach of Stanford University's powerhouse men's tennis team.

1. Hit the spot. You need to beat the ball to the place you want to make contact. Turn your right hand counterclockwise one-eighth of a turn over from your forehand grip. (Your palm should rest diagonally across the top of the handle.) Hold the throat of the racket lightly with your left hand. Spread the fingers of your right hand well apart.

2. Stay loose. Take a small step to the side with your left foot, and pivot on your right foot so that the back of your right shoulder faces the net. Maintaining a relaxed right arm, bring the racket head back along your waist and slightly behind your body. Don't tense up; you'll lose fluidity, and your powerful swing will turn into a feeble poke.

3. Collect power. Shift your weight onto your right foot, and drop the racket head below the height of the ball. Your knees should be bent. Keep a firm wrist (a loose wrist results in the ball floating up with little power or accuracy) and swing the racket forward. Simultaneously drop your left hand from the racket throat. When the ball rises to the level of your waist, hit it. Try to make contact with the outside edge of the ball so that you're driving it with as much leverage as possible. Maintaining a firm wrist, sweep the racket out and across your body, letting your body uncoil.

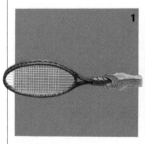
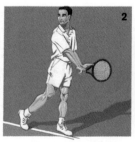
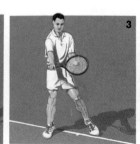
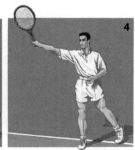

1 2 3 4

4. Finish with a flourish. At the end of the stroke, your right arm should be completely extended to the right side, and your wrist should be level with your eyes. Also, make sure the head of the racket is above your wrist. Your weight should be almost entirely on your right foot. Stand tall and relaxed, at least until the next shot.

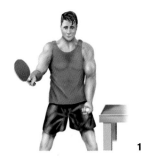

1

PING-PONG

How to Serve an Ace

Any activity that involves a paddle is bound to get nasty. Sean O'Neill, two-time Ping-Pong Olympian and five-time national singles champion, shows us how to deliver the most lethal serve in table tennis: the high toss. If you give it enough spin, it'll slice past your opponent like a curveball. If you don't, well, let's just say you'd better duck.

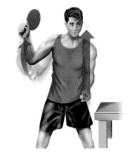

2

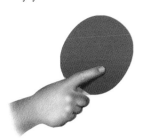

1. Get set. Stand at the far left of the table, with your left hip about 6 inches away from the corner. (If you're a lefty, move to the right side of the table.) Hold the paddle with a handshake grip about waist high, and extend your index finger for extra control.

2. Fling the ball high. While holding the ball in your palm, flick your wrist to toss the ball at least 6 feet high (pros go for 15 feet). The higher it goes, the more spin it'll have off the paddle. As the ball rises, swing your paddle hand back until it's level with your shoulder.

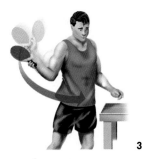

3

3. Twist and snap. When the ball is about 18 inches above the table, rotate your torso and swing the paddle down at the ball. Angle the paddle backward 20 degrees.

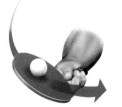

4

4. Slice it. At impact, snap your wrist forward to slice the underside of the ball. Giving it backspin will make it bounce unpredictably.

5. Follow through. Let your arm wind around your body. The perfect shot just clears the net and hits the direct center of your foe's court—at, oh, about 75 mph. Tip: If he tries to launch a blazing serve past you, keep your eyes focused just above center net. That'll give you a fighting chance of blocking it.

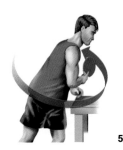

5

VOLLEYBALL

How to Jump Serve

A foolproof way to win at volleyball? Don't volley. If you learn how to deliver a jump serve, you'll drill the ball into the ground before the other team can react, says pro player Brian Lewis. Here's how he does it.

1. Line up the approach. Starting 6 feet behind the line, cradle the ball with both hands. Take four baby steps forward, crouching low to prepare for an explosive jump.

2. Toss it high. On step four, toss the ball with your right hand (or left for lefties, as shown) 6 feet above your head, 2 feet in front of you.

3. Put a spring in your step. Drive your arms back and up, jumping explosively off both feet, like Superman.

4. Cock your gun. Place your striking hand (palm open) behind your head at a 90-degree angle; point your other arm directly at the lofting ball. Arch your back.

5. Fire away. Blast your striking hand forward, hitting the top half of the ball, while plunging your other arm down. On the follow-through, point your striking arm where your meteor should land: center, far back.

MOUNTAIN BIKING

How to Execute a Pendulum Turn

Bo and Luke Duke made U-turns look so easy. But try their approach—hard braking, sharp turning—on a mountain bike and we'll read about you in the newspaper the next morning. You need finesse to nail a U-turn in the woods, explains George Clark, an expert racer. Practice in a grassy field, not on a tree-lined trail.

1. Approach the turn. Stop pedaling. Come off the seat 2 or 3 inches, knees bent, eyes focused, body upright. Lean forward.

2. Lift off. Squeeze the front brake so the rear wheel comes off the ground. Keep the pedals level.

3. Yank. Twist your head and upper body in the direction that you're turning. Then yank the handlebars so the rear end of the bike follows.

4. Push on. As the rear wheel lands, straighten out the handlebars and sit back; start pedaling to keep momentum.

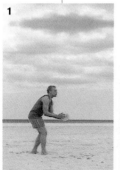
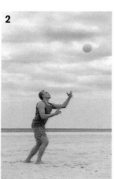
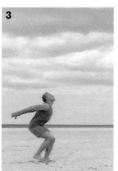
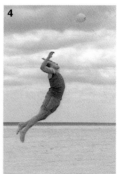
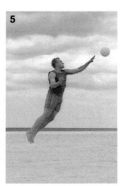

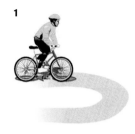
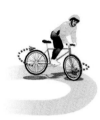
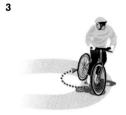
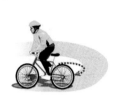

BASEBALL

How to Throw a Knuckler

So your fastball isn't what it used to be. It happens to all of us, well, except for Roger Clemens. Solution: Learn a new pitch. Bryan Mitchell, a two-time MVP in Amateur Softball Association tournaments, explains how to throw a dancing, wobbling knuckleball. (Lefties should reverse these instructions.)

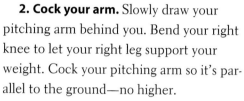

1. Get a grip. Keep your pinkie and thumb straight while gripping the ball with three knuckles along the laces, as shown.

2. Cock your arm. Slowly draw your pitching arm behind you. Bend your right knee to let your right leg support your weight. Cock your pitching arm so it's parallel to the ground—no higher.

3. Step forward. Swing your pitching arm forward, keeping it straight, in a smooth, underhand motion. As you do, take a 3-foot stride with your left foot.

4. Push the ball out. Release the ball by "pushing" it so that it doesn't spin. This takes practice. Don't flick your wrist or let the ball roll off your palm. If the ball has any sort of regular rotation, you're doing it wrong. But if the batter, catcher, and umpire all look perplexed, you're doing it right.

BY TREVOR THIEME

Best in Snow

Six sports you must try
this winter

Imagine this: It's the morning after a whiteout, and you're the first one off the chair. There's a virgin landscape of lush powder ahead of you, ripe for the plundering, and you've got two choices: Shred like a madman all day long and collapse into the hot tub, spent and stronger for it. Or start sucking wind after a couple of runs, fold like a hotel maid, and sulk in said hot tub until your fingers resemble giant, fleshy raisins.

You picked the first one, right? Then read on: Avalanche-inducing runs aren't built in a day. Follow the training tips we've assembled and you'll not only shred the slopes but yourself, too.

Snowshoeing

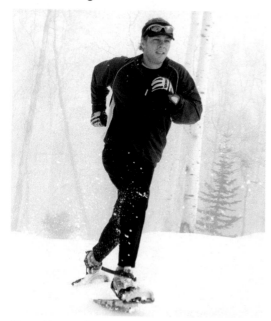

Steve Nyman Speed comes easily for this downhill skier, but not when he's strapped into a set of snowshoes, which he uses for training. The blizzard beaters helped him earn his first full-season World Cup berth last winter.

Why do it: Snowshoeing blasts your quadriceps, abdominals, and hip flexors—the latter get hit hard because snowshoes force you to walk with a funny-looking waddle. The sport also delivers a lot of bang for the cardiovascular buck: "Power walking 3 miles in snowshoes is the equivalent of doing 10 miles in sneakers," says Mike Bucek of the US Snowshoe Association. "The endurance it requires is really shocking."

The burn: 650 calories per hour

How to prep: "All of your power comes from your midsection," says Bucek. "So you'll need strong core muscles to keep your balance on soft snow." Start by spending 30 minutes, twice a week, on a stairclimber or cycling machine to help your feet get used to carrying the extra weight of snowshoes.

Next, work the exercises below into your routine. They're from Maureen Madden, CSCS, a physical therapist with The Stone Clinic, a rehabilitation center in San Francisco that specializes in sports medicine.

LUNGE ROTATIONS

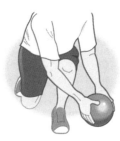

This exercise hits your quads and hip flexors, and conditions your body to handle steep hills and deep snow. Hold a medicine ball in both hands and take large strides across the floor. Keep your back straight but slightly inclined, and reach down to the outside of your front foot with the ball with each step. Make sure to rotate at your hip and keep your front foot flat (don't roll your ankle). Do three sets of 15 to 20 steps.

HIGH STEPPING

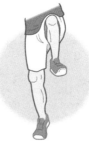

This exercise targets the calves, deltoids, hip flexors, and abdominals. Hold a medicine ball above your head and take high steps down a hall, rising up on your toes as if going for a layup. Again, three sets of 15 to 20 steps should do the trick.

Where to go: Anywhere, really. Local parks, golf courses, and even beaches (if you live in a temperate climate) are great places to start. Many of the nation's top ski resorts have snowshoe trails as well. In the Northeast, the Sunday River Cross Country Center in Maine (sundayriverinn.com) boasts more than 7 miles of trails that wind through woods and up nearby Barker Mountain. Out west, the new Nordic Center at the Resort at Squaw Creek in California (squaw.com) offers 12 miles of groomed trails that traverse the Squaw Valley meadow and surrounding hillside.

Downhill Skiing

Why do it: "Downhill skiing is one of the best outdoor sports for developing cardiovascular fitness," says Kevin Stone, MD, of The Stone Clinic. "You work the entire body." There's also an altitude effect, says Andy Walshe, sports science director for the US Ski Team. "High elevations place a heavy load on the respiratory system."

The burn: 350 calories per hour

How to prep: Cardio is crucial. And terrain changes at high and low speeds require

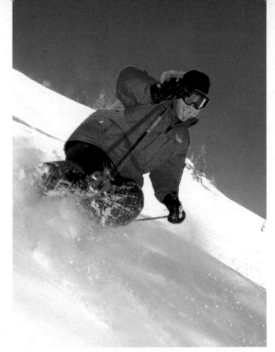

T.J. Lanning A knee blowout curtailed this US Ski Team member's rookie season, but he bounced back in 2004, winning the first World Cup time trial event of the season.

balance and coordination, which means you'll need strong abdominal and core muscles to keep your upper body taut while your legs power through each turn. Choose cross-training exercises that emphasize balance, short bursts of energy, and edge-to-edge movements, such as inline skating, mountain biking, skateboarding, or ice-skating. Once you acquire a strong aerobic foundation, start targeting the muscles you'll use with the following exercises.

PEAK
performance

May I Have This Dance?
Cross-train with your next date. Swedish researchers found that 12 weeks of dance training improved skiers' joint mobility, range of hip motion, and spinal flexibility. The subjects also experienced 67 percent less back pain after the training. According to the study, any type of dance that forces you to balance can help. The skiers in the study performed modern dance, jazz dance, or ballet.

THE SHREDDER
It hits the quads and glutes and simulates being on a ski edge, which helps tone the smaller support muscles that keep you balanced. Place a gym ball against a

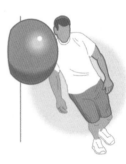

wall or post and lean into it with your right shoulder. Next, do a single-leg squat, being careful not to let your knee travel in front of your toes as you bend. Do three sets of 10 to 15 repetitions with each leg.

AROUND-THE-WORLD LUNGE

This is great for building leg strength and balance. Stand with your feet hip-width apart and hold dumbbells at your sides. Step backward with your right leg to 6 o'clock until your right knee is just above the floor and your left thigh is parallel to the floor. Keep your left knee over your toes. Push back to the starting position and repeat, this time stepping to 5 o'clock, but keeping your toes pointed straight ahead. Move counterclockwise until you reach 12 o'clock. Now switch legs and move clockwise from 6 o'clock to 12, hitting each hour along the way.

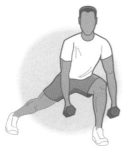

THE THROWER

This exercise is great for strengthening your core muscles and developing balance. Attach a sport cord to something above shoulder-level behind you, hold the other end in your right hand, and stand on your left leg. Rapidly pull the cord down and across your body as if throwing a fastball. Repeat 20 to 30 times, and switch sides. Do two sets with each hand.

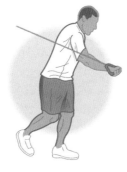

Where to go: Everyone has a favorite hill, but few rival the accessible terrain, vertical expanse, and rustic backcountry nooks and crannies of Whistler and Blackcomb in British Columbia (whistler-blackcomb.com).

You could spend an entire vacation exploring the 200-plus miles of combined trails—spread across 11 square miles—and never ski the same slope twice (unless, of course, you wanted to). Best of all, there's powder galore in the adjacent backcountry bowls and slopes.

Speed Skating

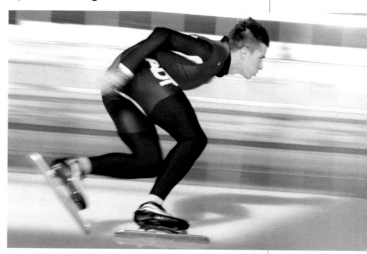

Kip Carpenter moved from the short to the long track 5 years ago. It paid off quickly: He struck bronze in the 500-meter at the 2002 Winter Olympics in Salt Lake City.

Why do it: It's low impact, compared with the other sports here. "You're not pounding the ground," explains Jack Mortell, short track coordinator for the US Speed Skating Association. "You're gliding into it." But low impact doesn't mean low benefit. It provides an excellent cardio workout and hammers just about every muscle in the legs, especially the quads, glutes, and hip abductors, which control the side-to-side movement of each stroke. What's more, speed skating places a strong emphasis on the abdominals, which are critical for maintaining balance and holding the crouched position.

The burn: 400 to 500 calories per hour

How to prep: Inline skating is hands down the best way to get in shape for speed skating; it uses essentially the same muscles and provides a great cardio pump. Mortell also recommends practicing your form in front of a mirror with a slide board (a shiny composite with foam bumpers on both ends). But if you're looking for more targeted exercises, try these.

MONSTER WALK

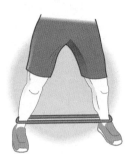

This exercise works your hip abductors. Wrap a tight resistance band around both ankles, keeping your feet shoulder-width apart, knees bent. Step sideways across the room with toes pointed straight ahead or slightly inward. Do 10 steps to the right, 10 to the left, and repeat 3 times.

LATERAL LEAP INTERVALS

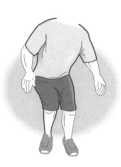

This drill develops leg strength and explosive power. Use two parallel strips of tape to establish your jump parameters on the floor. Leap sideways and land outside the far piece of tape. When you jump back, stay inside the near piece. Do five to seven 30-second intervals, then three 1-minute intervals.

Where to go: There are only five long tracks in the United States: Lake Placid, New York; Roseville, Minnesota; Butte,

Montana; Milwaukee; and Salt Lake City. But most hockey rinks transform into short tracks on occasion—there's a good chance you can get ice time at a local university in the northern half of the country. For more on recreational speed skating, check out www.tryspeedskating.com.

Snowboarding

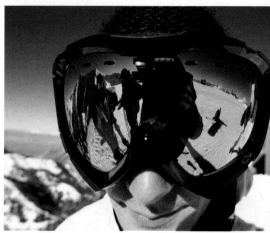

George Oakley took first place in the Slope Style competition at the North American Snowboarding Championships in 2004, and third place overall in the Vans Triple Crown rankings.

Why do it: Whether you're ripping a half-pipe or just cruising downhill, snowboarding provides both a monster cardio workout and a serious muscle-building pump. If you really want to push your aerobic threshold, spend a day at the terrain park. "A study a few years back tracked snowboarders in the half-pipe," says Ron Kipp, a consultant to the Norwegian Ski Team. "Between performing tricks and hiking up it, they were operating near their physiological limits." You'll work the same muscles snowboarding as you would while alpine skiing—calves, quads, and hamstrings—but in snowboarding, the abdominals become particularly important for maintaining good form, as the boarder has to counter-rotate his upper body to control each turn.

The burn: 350 calories per hour

How to prep: The best way is to practice a crossover sport like surfing or skateboarding, which utilizes the same balance muscles and movement patterns. But because snowboarding and skateboarding promote greater muscle development in the rear leg—a consequence of using it to ambulate across flat ground—it's important to exercise each leg individually to maintain a balance between them. (An imbalance can lead to lower back problems because your hamstrings connect directly to your pelvis.) Use the following exercises to do just that.

SINGLE-LEG SQUATS ON A FOAM ROLL

Besides strengthening your hammies, glutes, and quads, this exercise will help you develop the heel-edge and toe-edge balance needed for snowboarding. Stand with one leg

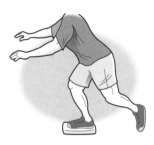

on a piece of foam roll, move your other leg back (but keep it off the ground) for balance, and squat while reaching forward with both arms. Do two to three sets of 15 repetitions on each leg.

SINGLE-LEG STANDING REACH-DOWNS

This exercise targets single-leg balance, glute muscle strengthening, and trunk stability. Stand on your left leg and bend your right knee about 45 degrees. Then, holding a 3- to 8-pound dumb-

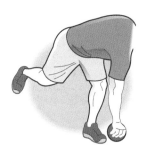

bell or weighted ball in your right hand, reach down and touch the ground near your left ankle. Repeat 15 times, then switch both your foot and your hand. Complete two sets on each side.

Where to go: Great terrain parks are hard to come by. We like California's Mammoth Mountain (mammothmountain.com), which includes zones for all skill levels. Mammoth also has 40 rails, 50 jumps, and a monstrous half-pipe with 18-foot walls spread across three separate terrain parks.

Cross-Country Skiing

Why do it: Cross-country skiing is one of those rare exercises that enlist every muscle. Diagonal strides rip the quads, glutes, and hamstrings; poling pumps the lats, triceps, and biceps. The abs also get hit hard, as they stabilize and propel the body through each stride. "You get more bang for your buck than any other winter sport," says Kipp. "If you want to burn calories, this is the way to do it."

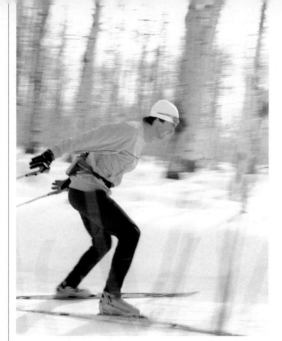

Johnny Spillane At age 22, he became the first American ever to win a world championship gold medal in the Nordic Combined, a cross-training sport that pairs ski jumping with cross-country skiing.

The burn: 750 calories per hour

How to prep: Leg strength and cardio endurance are key, so the best way to train is to run—as far and as often as possible. Also, roller-skating helps leg muscles prepare for side-to-side movement. Try the following strength exercises to increase power and endurance.

THE REACHER

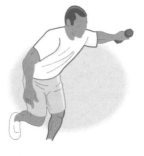

It improves balance, glute strength, and trunk stability. Stand on your left leg, holding a 5- to 8-pound dumbbell in your left hand, arms straight. Then slowly raise your left arm so it's parallel to the floor. Pause 3 seconds, then lower it back to your side. Switch sides. Do two sets of 10 reps on each side.

SINGLE-LEG REACH DIPS

These develop endurance and strength in your hammies, glutes, and quads. Face a post or wall two paces away. Stand on your right leg, then lean forward and touch the wall at waist height with your hands. Repeat 10 to 15 times in 1 minute. Aim for three sets on each leg.

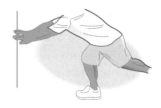

SINGLE-LEG SPORT-CORD PULLBACK

It simultaneously works the muscles you need for skating and poling and improves balance. Attach two sport cords to something sturdy 10 feet in front of you and hold one in each hand. Stand on your right leg, then squat while pulling back the right cord. Switch sides. Do three sets of 15 reps on each leg.

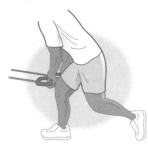

Where to go: Your backyard is fine, but if you're a beginner, start on groomed trails—there's less plowing and more gliding, making it easier to learn. Check skisite.com for trails near you.

Ice Climbing

Why do it: Ice climbing provides an excellent full-body workout, focusing on three areas: legs, arms, and torso. Your quads and glutes get hit as you slide your body up the ice, and your calves get a workout as you balance on ice-anchored crampons. Meanwhile, your rotator cuffs, biceps, and triceps get hammered as you swing your ice ax and pull your body from placement to placement. And your midsection gets pumped from keeping your body stable and your movements coordinated.

The burn: 400 to 600 calories per hour

How to prep: "Ice climbing is sort of like boxing," explains Peter Athans, who, with seven summits, has conquered Everest more than any other non-Sherpa climber. "It's brutal. To train for it, you have to do just about everything." He means a heavy dose of cardio—cycling, swimming, and running—and plenty of weight training.

Here's how to get started.

RESISTANCE TRAINING WITH A SPORT CORD

This is a great way to condition your arms for the whacking and hacking of ice climbing. Attach one end of the cord to a sturdy anchor 10 feet away, holding the other end with 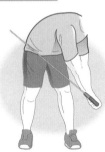 both hands. Start chopping as if you're holding an ice ax. Switch hands and repeat. Start with 2-minute intervals, building the intensity and length of your sets as you get better.

PRONE ON BALL REACHES

These are excellent for strengthening your rotator cuffs. Position yourself facedown on a 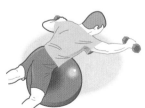 gym ball, holding a weight in each hand at ear level. Reach forward one arm at a time, performing two sets of 15 reaches with each arm.

BODY SCISSORS

This exercise strengthens your abs and upper body while improving balance. Place your hands on a bench and toes on a gym ball, keeping your back 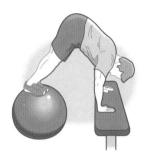 flat. Use your abs to pull your body up into a pike position, then slowly reverse. Perform two sets of 5 to 10 reps.

DUMBBELL PULLOVER EXTENSION

This develops your upper back and triceps, preventing arm fatigue. Lie faceup with dumbbells held straight over your chest. Keep your biceps steady and drop the weights until your elbows hit 90 degrees. Then lower your arms so your elbows hit your ears. Do three sets of 10 to 15 reps.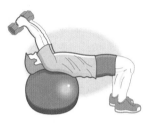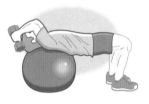

Where to go: The premier US destination for ice climbing is Ouray, Colorado. Ten years ago, three climbers began tapping local water pipes, diverting the flow over the edge of nearby Uncompahgre Gorge. The result: instant waterfalls and the country's first and only ice park (ourayicepark.com). Best of all: It's free. Athans also likes Lake Willoughby, Vermont, which features some of the longest steep ascents in the Northeast, and North Conway, New Hampshire, revered for the sheer variety of terrain.

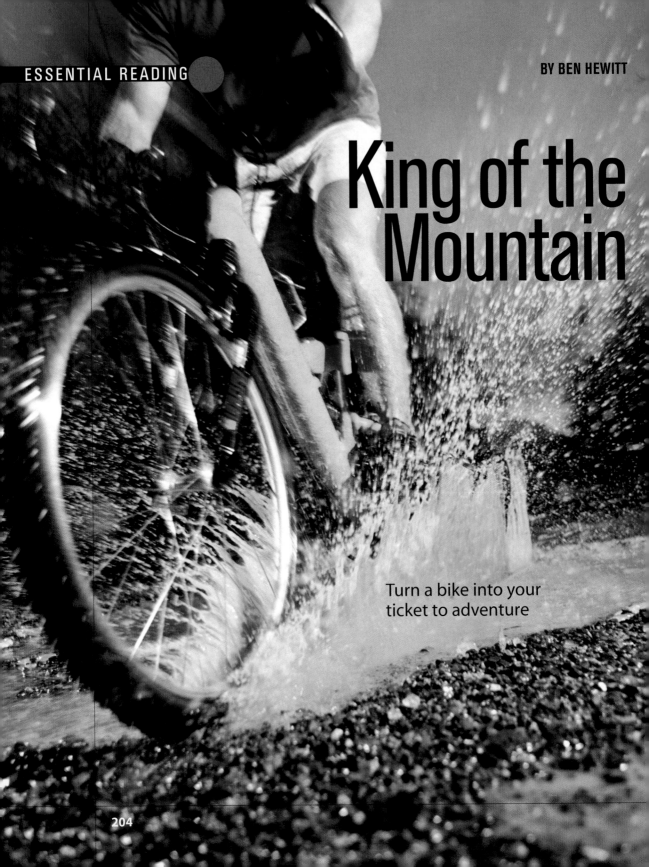

BY BEN HEWITT

King of the Mountain

Turn a bike into your
ticket to adventure

ilip Meirhaeghe isn't used to standing still. But high on a hill overlooking Quebec's St. Lawrence River, on a narrow ribbon of muddy trail spiked with snot-slick rocks, the best mountain biker in the world has stopped pedaling.

In fact, he's hovering over me, inspecting a flap of skin ripped from my right knee courtesy of a rain-slicked root. "You have too much air pressure in your tires," he says, with an I've-seen-worse shrug. He gives my rear tire a cantaloupe squeeze, then wheels around and disappears into the brush.

It's choice nuggets of wisdom like this (and maybe his mammoth thighs, zeppelin-size lungs, and years in the saddle) that made Meirhaeghe the 2003 cross-country world champion and a former kingpin on the balls-to-the-wall downhill circuit. They also make him the perfect two-wheeled trail guide for the bruising, top-notch course I've only just begun to tackle.

Meirhaeghe's mission: to shred my riding style in search of the most common mistakes that you'll make on the trail and the easy fixes that you, I, and even some of his rivals could benefit from. Listen up—or learn the hard way.

Trail Trick #1: Deflate Your Tires

Make sure your tires are primed to handle off-road terrain. At 45 psi, mine were overinflated—pumped for a paved bike path, where a stiff, unforgiving tire makes you more efficient. (Road-bike tires are often inflated to more than 100 psi.) At Meirhaeghe's suggestion, I drop my pressure to 30 psi and

notice the difference right away. My tires envelop the terrain instead of riding on top of it, and cushion blows on the tough stuff. The hidden benefit: You're less likely to blow a tire when you slam into protruding rocks.

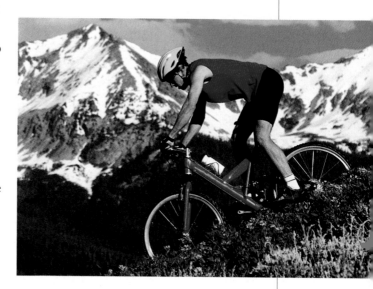

Trail Trick #2: Don't Steer

Your bike has shocks, so use them. Cautiously picking your way between obstacles will only slow you down and mess with your center of gravity. "The straightest line is the fastest and the easiest," says Meirhaeghe, before making a neat bell curve over a giant boulder blocking our path while I grab a fistful of brakes and zigzag my way around it. Practice scaling smaller roots and rocks first, keeping your eyes at least a dozen feet ahead on the trail. Then move on to larger obstacles, such as timbers or fallen trees placed midtrail as speed bumps or "stunts." See "Steal These Moves" on page 206 for the technique.

Steal These Moves

And look like a pro

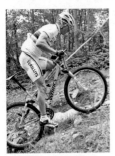

Going Up

On steep climbs, the goal is to keep your front wheel grounded without losing rear traction. Position your torso over the handlebar, but keep your hips low and back so the rear wheel maintains its grip. On extremely steep hills, try sitting on the tip of your saddle—but first make sure you've got a sturdy pair of bike shorts, such as the Nema Crown Jewel ($90; nema-usa.com).

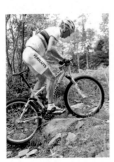

Getting Over

Sticks and stones can, and will, make splinters of your bones if you don't learn the art of quick weight transfer. As you reach an obstacle, lean back and pull up slightly to lift the bike's front wheel. Then shift your weight forward immediately, push down lightly on the handlebar, and "lift" the rear wheel with your legs.

Coming Down

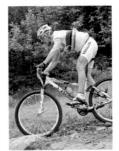

Tense up and you'll wipe out. Keep a relaxed and ready posture—knees and elbows bent to help absorb bumps, eyes ahead—and you'll be able to dodge or absorb any nasty surprises. On extremely steep descents, straighten your arms and move your butt behind the saddle to take weight off the front wheel.

Trail Trick #3: Shhh!

"Be one with your bike," Meirhaeghe says, waxing *Caddyshack* during our first steep drop, a rubble-strewn wasteland leading down into a valley. "Try to ride so that it is as quiet as possible." When your bike makes noise, he explains, you're losing speed because you're hitting obstacles or shifting incorrectly. And, sure enough, Meirhaeghe's bike is ninja-silent as he whizzes down the trail, while mine clanks and rattles with all the stealth of an Abrams tank. The key is keeping your arms and legs loose, using your body as a second set of shocks to absorb whatever the ground dishes out. The ground comes up, you crouch down—and your center of gravity stays put. Keep your joints bent slightly, ready to flex with the bike. You'll not only retain better control of your ride and prevent yourself from being bucked off by a dirt speed bump, but you'll also be microadjusting your balance to the terrain, making last-second swerves around boulders less precarious—anything to stay in the saddle.

Trail Trick #4: Use Wheel Power

Cranking hard over slick rocks and roots can cause you to spin out, cutting your speed, traction, and forward momentum. If you can't make it up a hill on oomph alone, put the pedal down when it counts—on dirt. "Power the pedals before the root or rock, then let up as your rear wheel rolls over. Then start pedaling hard again," Meirhaeghe advises. Use your head before you lose your head of steam: If you see a steep ascent

Street Smarts

How to apply your newfound skills to the concrete jungle

The sidewalk isn't much different from the dirt track: The techniques are the same, only the terrain has changed. That's why you'll want a ride that's more pavement-friendly—solid mountain-bike frame, road tires, no rear shocks to suck up your pedaling power and slow you down. We like the Marin Point Reyes ($900; marinbikes.com), which is equal parts ruggedness and road manners. Lieutenant Tom Woods, an instructor for the International Mountain Bike Police Association, explains how to translate off-road skills into urban assault tactics.

The skill: Screeching halt

The threat: Car doors, wayward hot-dog carts

The how-to: "A wheel with no weight has no traction," says Woods. "Shift your weight back as you brake and you'll be able to use more braking power without getting bucked." Level your pedals. Scoot your butt to the back edge of the saddle. Straighten your arms, but don't lock your elbows. Bend your knees to act as shock absorbers. Hit the rear brake first, then the front brake, hard.

The skill: Obstacle climbing

The threat: Curbs

The how-to: "You want to use leverage instead of brute force to get up and over," Woods says. Approach the curb perpendicularly with your pedals at two o'clock and eight o'clock, your stronger foot forward and up. Click into a gear that's one or two harder than you'd normally ride. About a foot before the curb, push down on the pedal for oomph as you pull up on the bar (like popping a partial wheelie). Once your front wheel is up, shift your weight forward to pull the rear wheel over.

The skill: Kamikaze descent

The threat: Stairs

The how-to: "If you get used to allowing momentum to have its way, stairs will smooth out," says Woods. Shift into a higher gear to increase chain tension so the chain won't pop off. Feather your brakes, if needed, to adjust your speed. Pick a line that's perpendicular to the stairs, level your pedals, and move your butt behind the rear of the saddle. Flex your arms and legs.

The skill: Big air

The threat: Railroad tracks, manholes, potholes, jumping rooftop to rooftop

The how-to: Maintain a straight line and level your pedals at least three bike lengths before the obstacle. A foot before, compress your body, flexing your arms and bending your knees as you bring your torso down almost to parallel to the ground. Then spring up, lifting the front and rear wheels off the ground at the same time.

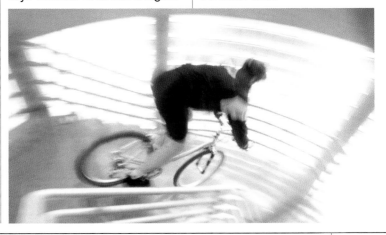

looming on the horizon, kick in some extra legwork. You'll need it on the way up.

Trail Trick #5: Flex Your Abs

Descending a steep hill can be risky business, as aggressive braking can cause the front wheel to lock up and skid, especially on slick trails. The front brake is where you'll find 80 percent of your stopping power, so you can't ignore your left hand altogether. But turn your hands into a makeshift antilock brake system and you'll keep control of your descent. Start to brake with your rear pads, then add in as much front as you can. Feather the brakes immediately if the front wheel begins to slide or, worse, lock up. And don't forget to shift your weight backward to keep yourself on the right side of the handlebar. Practice braking on flat, dry ground first, and you'll get a feel for it without having to pick through grass for your missing teeth.

Trail Trick #6: Go Long

Hard riding is sort of like tequila: A little is a very good thing, but too much and you'll find yourself on the rocks. "You shouldn't do it more than two times each week," says Meirhaeghe. Even if you're riding only twice a week, make sure one of those days is a long ride at a comfortable pace. Long rides build endurance, the secret weapon of pro riders—it ensures that they always have a burst of speed left in reserve, even after a full day of riding, for attacking that last runoff chute, slippery boulder, or race to the finish.

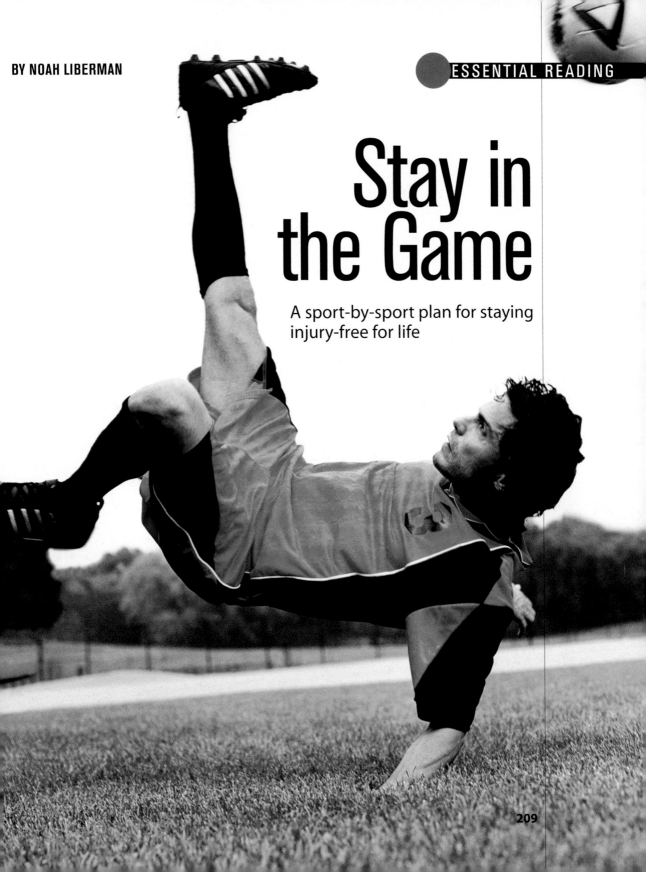

BY NOAH LIBERMAN

Stay in the Game

A sport-by-sport plan for staying injury-free for life

We know a guy—let's call him Bill—whose basketball game has gone like this:

Age 8: Finally reaches hoop with ball.

Age 12: Starts to get good.

Age 17: Stars on high school basketball team.

Age 20: Still turns heads in college pickup games.

Ages 24 to 34: Focuses on career.

Age 35: Can't hit a 3 to save his life; knees are killing him; periodically throws out left shoulder; vertical leap is a lean.

Don't let this happen to you. People like Bill will tell you that the problem with sports is that they're designed for young people. To which we respond: So stay young.

It's not only possible, but we've laid out the plan right here. The trick is getting started now, systematically strengthening the body parts most battered by your favorite activity. The other key is not taking your eye off the ball: If you step away from the game for too long, it might become harder to get back into it after a certain age.

We're not talking about some metaphysical fountain of youth, either. No, this is straight sports medicine. Do the exercises recommended in the following pages for your sport and you'll stay in the game until the big head coach in the sky benches you for good.

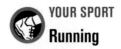

YOUR SPORT
Running

Where it gets you: In both knees

How to stay in the game: Go faster for shorter distances.

Your first instinct as a runner is probably to go as far as possible, even if it means a slow pace. But that's backward, says Bill Mallon, MD, an orthopedic surgeon and a consultant to US Olympic teams. Going longer and slower only makes you a worse runner because your tired body can't maintain proper form. This problem is compounded by thickly padded motion-control shoes, which are designed to make those long, sloppy runs more comfortable. They control the movement of your feet and ankles, so your knees take more of a beating.

Instead, improve your running technique by going faster for shorter distances. "You can't run fast with terrible biomechanics," Dr. Mallon says. Short, fast runs will improve your form—specifically, how quickly

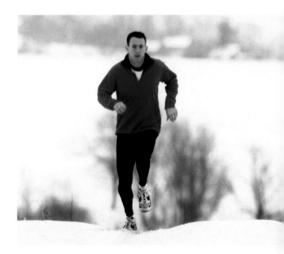

your feet lift off the ground after striking it. The faster your feet leave the ground, the less impact your knees will have to absorb.

Next time you run, go for 30 minutes and determine how far you went. Then, once a week for the next 4 weeks, try to cover the same distance in less time. After those 4 weeks, pick a slightly longer distance, establish how long it takes you to run it, and then try to beat that time for the following 4 weeks. Eventually, you should be able to do all distances faster and with better form.

Bonus Running Tip: Now that you're running shorter distances faster, wear a pair of racing flats instead of running shoes. Flats are simple, light shoes with little padding—basically, track shoes without spikes. You'll feel your feet in action and be able to tell when your form isn't right. You can buy racing flats at any sporting goods store with a specialty running section.

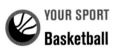

YOUR SPORT
Basketball

Where it gets you: In both ankles
How to stay in the game: Stretch and strengthen the muscles around your ankles.

Most pro basketball players sprain their ankles more often than they nail groupies. We've all seen the slow-motion replays and watched the players mouth obscenities. "Basketball players are always coming down on other guys' feet," says Nicholas DiNu-

bile, MD, team orthopedist for the Philadelphia 76ers.

When this happens, the natural inclination of your ankle is to roll outward. The ligaments in your ankle are quickly stretched beyond their natural length, and inflammation ensues.

That's not the worst of it: After the pain and swelling abate, the ligaments in your ankle can remain at 80 percent of their preinjury strength for a long time. That dramatically increases the chance that you'll have more sprains, which creates psychological barriers: If you know you have gimpy gams, you'll play more tentatively.

For rehabilitation or prevention of ankle problems, try the following three exercises, which are illustrated in "Your Lifetime Warranty Starts Here" on page 212. Each can be done on the court while you're waiting for your pickup team to join the fray—or in your living room as you watch the Final Four.

Calf stretches. Tight calves increase the chance of a sprain, Dr. DiNubile says. There are two major stretches—straight knee and bent knee—each working a different part of the calf muscle. Make sure you hold for at least 30 seconds.

Tendon strengtheners. Place a circular piece of exercise tubing around the balls of both feet (a bungee cord works just fine, too). Sit on a chair with your heels on the floor and your toes off the ground. Rotate both feet outward, away from each other and against the resistance.

Your Lifetime Warranty Starts Here

Spot the icon for your sport and get to work

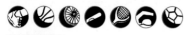

ABDOMINALS

Do three to five sets of 15 to 20 repetitions.

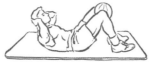

BALANCE DRILL

Hold for as long as you can on each leg; repeat three times with both legs.

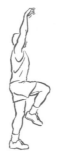

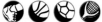

CALF STRETCHES

Try both types, holding each for 30 seconds. Do each stretch three times per leg.

  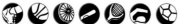

GLUTEALS

Do one to three sets of six to eight repetitions with each leg.

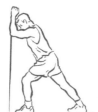 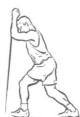

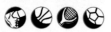

ANKLES

Do three to five sets of 10 repetitions.

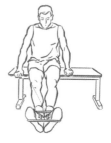

ARMS

Do three sets of five rotations with each arm. Build up to three sets of 15.

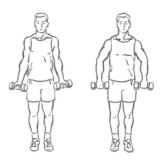

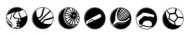

LOWER BACK

Hold for 15 seconds per repetition. Work up to one or two sets of eight repetitions.

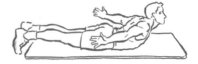

ROTATOR CUFF

Do three to five sets of 10 to 15 repetitions of each exercise, using light weight for all.

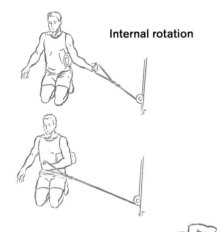

Internal rotation

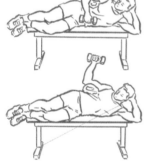

External rotation

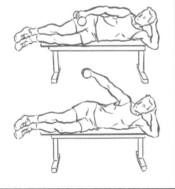

Abduction

Balance drills. Close your eyes and try to balance on one foot. Shoot imaginary baskets or make other motions to add to the challenge. Try it standing on a short length of a two-by-four. "It feels silly, but it improves your balance and fine-tunes the condition of your ankles," Dr. DiNubile says.

Bonus Basketball Tip: Replace your shoes when the outer edge of the heel begins to wear down. A worn heel makes it too easy for an ankle to roll over and result in a sprain.

YOUR SPORT
Bicycling

Where it gets you: Knees, back, hips, feet
How to stay in the game: Your bike must match your body.

Here's how to size up your bike.

Frame. Stand with your bare feet 6 inches apart. Have your girlfriend measure your inseam from crotch to floor. (Not dating anyone? Ask an intern.) Multiply

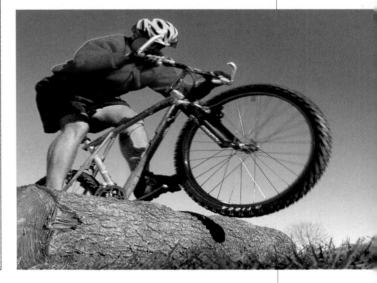

your inseam by 0.65. That's the frame size you need.

Seat height. At the bottom of your pedal stroke, your knee should be slightly bent.

Saddle tilt. You want it level or turned up slightly in front.

If you're going to be doing a lot of riding, other variables come into play. Your height,

PAINkiller

Sit It Out

While I was playing soccer, my lower back tightened up. Two weeks later, it still hurts—especially after I've been sitting for a while. What did I do?
                                                  N.B., Carmel, Indiana

Any kind of lunging or twisting motion can strain your back muscles. It's also possible you've pulled the paraspinal muscle, commonly injured during kicking sports. If you feel any tingling in your legs or feet, you need to see a doctor to rule out nerve damage. Otherwise, take it easy because the muscles in the back take several weeks to rehab. And ice the area after any exercise.

the length of your arms, and the amount of arch in your feet could affect your comfort and how long you ride injury-free.

You attain that marriage of man and bike by pedaling over to the best bike shop in town, one that uses either the Ben Serotta Size Cycle system or the Ergo-Fit Method from Bicycle Fitting Systems, suggests Andy Pruitt, EdD, a sports medicine specialist in Boulder, Colorado. You'll pay between $50 and $125 for a fitting, which takes about 30 to 45 minutes. For the location of a Ben Serotta system near you, check out serotta.com; for Ergo-Fit, see bicyclefit.com.

Bonus Bicycling Tip: Build your abs and lower-back muscles separately. Bicycling gives

you a very strong lower body from pedaling, and somewhat strong arms and upper back from pulling on the handlebars during climbs. "But your core is surprisingly weak," says Pruitt. So you're a fit guy everywhere except the part of your body where you're most likely to be injured while working around the house or playing other sports. And an injured back will make cycling uncomfortable and cut your endurance substantially. Avoid these problems by doing the exercises in "Your Lifetime Warranty Starts Here" on page 212.

YOUR SPORT
Soccer

Where it gets you: Ankles, knees, hips, lower back

How to stay in the game: Find a balance.

A soccer player kicks the ball with a motion that's forward and toward the midline of his body. This gives him inner thighs that could crack nuts (if he isn't careful) but relatively weak outer thighs and gluteals, says Rich Monis, former head athletic trainer for the Chicago Fire, a major league soccer team. This muscle imbalance can lead to chronic injuries in the lower back, hips, and knees.

Try the gluteal exercise on page 212. It requires balance, so the outer-hip muscles will work hard to stabilize your body.

Bonus Soccer Tip: The stronger your legs become, the more important it is to keep your abs and lower back correspondingly strong, Monis says. After you do the gluteal exercise, do our abdominal and lower-back exercises on page 212, too.

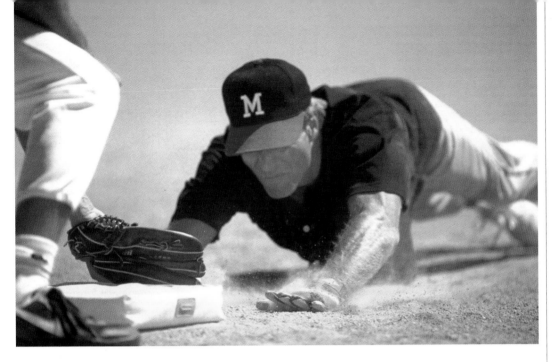

YOUR SPORT
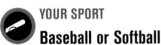
Baseball or Softball

Where it gets you: Shoulders and arms
How to stay in the game: Throw year-round.

Professional baseball pitchers know that throwing puts a tremendous strain on a person's arms, shoulders, and neck. The result could be anything from torn muscles in your rotator cuff to a broken arm.

To prevent this, chuck it around as often as possible during the off-season. Throw a minimum of once a week throughout the winter, even if it's just a quick, chilly game of catch, says Richard Ferkel, MD, an orthopedic surgeon in Van Nuys, California. Research shows that the humerus, or upper-arm bone, actually thickens and strengthens with consistent throwing, which keeps your rotator cuff strong and supple. The result is an arm and shoulder that won't snap during spring training.

You should also do the following baseball-friendly exercises in the weight room: wrist curls and extensions; biceps curls and triceps extensions; front and lateral raises for the deltoids; and forearm rotators, in which you hold a weight at the beginning position of a biceps curl, then simply rotate

PAINkiller

Elbowed Out
While throwing a baseball to my kids, I felt a searing pain on the inside of my elbow. What was that? And how can I keep it from happening again?
F.Y., Lynchburg, Virginia

The most common elbow injury is "pitcher's elbow," or elbow tendinitis. The tendon attaching the flexor muscles to the humerus bone (in your upper arm) can become inflamed as a result of repetitive motion or stress on the area from bad throwing form. (Don't feel bad; it even happens to the pros.) In the future, stretch your shoulders and elbows before getting out on the field. You can protect the joint by doing dumbbell curls to strengthen your forearms and biceps. And take it easy: Talent scouts aren't hanging out at your ball field.

your palms forward and back, which mimics the rotations of the throwing motion. (See "Your Life-time Warranty Starts Here" on page 212.) Start with light weights and higher repetitions.

Finally, to prevent the dreaded rotator-cuff tear, do the three rotator-cuff exercises we show as well. Do all these weight-room exercises twice a week.

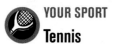

YOUR SPORT
Tennis

Where it gets you: Shoulders, elbows, calves

How to stay in the game: Strengthen your rotator cuffs.

The tennis serve may be the most unnatural motion an athlete can make. Not only does the serving motion itself render players susceptible to rotator-cuff tears, but the stress

on the shoulder and elbow is magnified by the stop-shock of a racket hitting the ball. That can produce tennis elbow, tendinitis in the shoulder, or both. Either injury makes playing tennis painful, if not impossible. It makes life in general kinda annoying as well.

The solution starts with the rotator-cuff exercises shown on page 213. Combine them with the arm and shoulder exercises that we suggest for baseball and softball players.

Next, check with a tennis pro to see if you're using the right racket and proper string tension for your body and the type of game you play, suggests Mark Kaufman, a physical therapist in Chicago and a consultant to World Team Tennis. And when you do buy a new racket, remember that you need a get-acquainted period. Each racket requires your body to make minute mechanical adjustments for each stroke. Give your muscles and connective tissues a week or two to adjust before you go out and play five sets.

And if you're injured? "Sometimes you have to eliminate a part of the game to aid recovery. You may have to forget serves or overhead shots for a few weeks until the inflammation dies down," Kaufman says.

Bonus tennis tip: Playing tennis also puts a lot of stress on your calves and, especially, your Achilles tendons. Quick starts, stops, and changes of direction put your Achilles at greater risk of rupture than most other

PAIN killer

Tackling Pain
My college football career beat me all to hell. Will using anti-inflammatory medications for the pain put me at risk of further injury when I play sports now?

A.I., Tulsa, Oklahoma

Taking Advil or Celebrex, or whatever works for you, is fine. The danger is overmedicating to the point that you do more damage because you can't feel enough pain while playing. Pain is your body's way of preventing injury. If you're hurting, it's a signal to take a time-out. Otherwise, enjoy playing.

sports, Kaufman notes. To help protect them, add the calf stretches on page 212 to your repertoire.

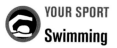

YOUR SPORT
Swimming

Where it gets you: In the shoulders
How to stay in the game: Add variety to your workouts.

Shoulder impingement sinks a lot of serious swimmers. Muscles and connective tissues inside the shoulder capsule swell up and rub against bone, which causes more swelling. The inflammation makes swimming painful—heck, it can even make the simple act of putting on a shirt excruciating. It also leads to scar-tissue buildup, which changes the way the muscles move and nerves react. Try this three-tiered strategy to keep inflammation from limiting your time in the pool.

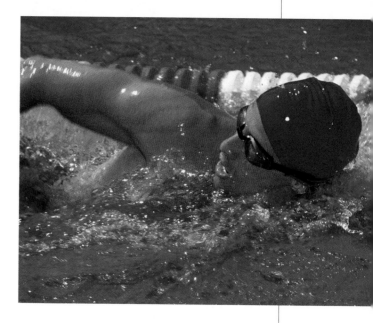

1. Incorporate a variety of strokes into each workout. Focusing on one stroke is a recipe for shoulder problems, so mix it up. The backstroke and breaststroke, for example, work your shoulder muscles very differently, giving them periodic R&R.

2. Add short bursts of faster swimming to some of your workouts. This not only forces your shoulder muscles to work at varying intensities, but it also makes you use fewer strokes per lap.

3. On dry land, do the rotator-cuff exercises shown on page 213.

Training Tips

Q **My knees take a pounding when I play sports. Any strategies to keep them healthy?**
P.P., FLINT, MICHIGAN

A Work on your landings. Whether you're jumping on a basketball court or bounding across a tennis court, your knees are at risk if you don't have the strength to decelerate the load—that load being you.

"I don't think there's enough emphasis placed on our ability to bring our bodies to a controlled stop," says Robert Dos Remedios, MS, CSCS, director of speed, strength, and conditioning at the

HOOPS

Give Your Game a Lift

It's a time-honored tradition for basketball players to blame lousy play on the weight lifting they recently did. That won't fly anymore. Researchers at Brigham Young University have shown that weight lifting doesn't hurt basketball performance. They found no difference in the vertical jump or shooting accuracy of 18 Division I basketball players whether or not the players did total-body workouts 6 hours prior to playing. "All energy systems should recover an hour or two after lifting," says Mandy Woolstenhulme, a PhD candidate and the lead study author. The key, she says, is to do a moderate-intensity workout so you don't incur muscle soreness. Lift harder on weeks when you don't play or during the off-season.

College of the Canyons. If you plan on doing any type of explosive training—the kind needed for most sports—make landings part of your workouts for at least a month, says Dos Remedios.

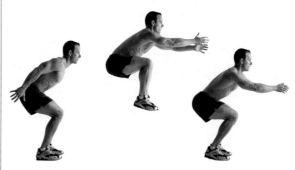

Between sets of squats or other leg exercises, do five jumps on a semisoft surface, like a rubber-matted area in your gym. Stand with your feet shoulder-width apart. Jump straight up. Then focus on landing with your knees bent, shoulders slightly forward, and butt and hips back. Try to land on the front two-thirds of your feet, with your heels just barely off the ground. Progress to tuck jumps: Bring your knees up high toward your chest to make it harder to stick the landings.

IN THE SWING OF THINGS

Q **My hip feels like it's going to pop out of place every time I swing a baseball bat. Do you have any idea why?**
A.W., ARLINGTON, VIRGINIA

A It's most likely some hip-joint instability or weakness of the muscles and soft tissues that make up the "hip girdle," the group of muscles around the

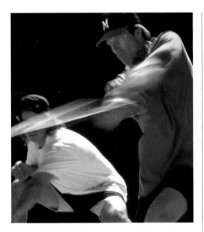

hip joint. Some people are born with a joint abnormality called hip dysplasia, and others simply have loose joints. It could also be a meniscus tear or damage to a tendon. If there's no pain, don't sweat it. Meanwhile, stop swinging for the fences. There's nothing wrong with hitting a solid double every once in a while.

WARMING UP

How should I adjust my workout to get ready for warm-weather sports like softball and golf?
Y.T., PISCATAWAY, NEW JERSEY

If you're ramping up for any activity that requires strenuous arm and shoulder work—throwing, swinging, even pulling ropes on a sailboat—you have to work your rotator cuffs. To do that, add to your workout the rotational pushup on a medicine ball.

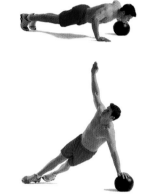

Get into a pushup position with your right hand on the floor and your left hand on a medicine ball. As you straighten your arms, lift your right hand off the floor and raise it until your arm points toward the ceiling. Keep your back straight and don't bend your knees—you want to make your left arm work harder to stabilize on the medicine ball. After a set of 8 to 10, switch arms and repeat.

CONTAINMENT POLICY

We always wore jocks in high school, but now most of my sports shorts have those built-in briefs. Is this enough protection?
M.L., PORTLAND, MAINE

Only you can tell. The purpose of jockstraps and sports shorts is more for containment than for support. If the shorts are enough to keep your equipment from excessive flopping—and you've experienced no pain—you're fine. One recommendation: If you're playing softball or other contact sports, wear a cup.

Hop to It

Strengthening your hips can help your hops. A study published in the *Journal of Strength and Conditioning Research* found that your hip extensors—mainly the hamstrings and gluteus maximus—are more responsible for jumping high than your calves, quads, or ankles are. The researchers measured the amount of muscle activity at the ankle, knee, and hip joints when men jumped low and when they jumped high. Activity levels remained the same at the ankles and knees for low jumps and high jumps, but were greater at the hip for the highest jumps, says lead author Adrian Lees, PhD. Target your hamstrings and glutes with squats, hamstring curls, and glute bridges.

Credits

Cover
© Darryl Estrine

Interior Photography
© Lori Adamski-Peek: pages iv (snowboarder), 196, 197, 198, 199, 200, 202
© Jack Affleck: page 191
© Steve Ballot: page 194
© Ondrea Barbe: pages 30, 64, 176
© Jim Baron: page 159 (mountain lion)
© Beth Bischoff: pages 50, 51, 52, 53, 59, 67, 68, 75, 76, 77, 79, 80, 81, 83, 91 (exercises), 97, 98, 99, 102, 104, 105, 106 (exercises), 107, 111, 112, 113, 116, 117, 118, 119 (exercises), 120, 123, 125, 126, 127, 130, 131, 132, 133 (exercises), 138, 139, 140, 141, 144, 145, 146, 147, 148, 149 (exercises), 155, 218, 219 (exercises)
© Brand X Pictures: page 175 (left)
© Corbis: pages iv (tennis), 70, 178, 205
© Tom Brakefield/Corbis: page 158
© Jim Erickson/Corbis: page 207
© Patrik Giardino/Corbis: page 204
© Uwe Walz/Corbis: page 159 (boar)
© Jim Zuckerman/Corbis: page 159 (bear)
© Richard Corman: pages 58, 84
© Tim Defrisco: page 179
© Digital Vision: page 187 (runner)
© Tom Dipace: page 183 (football players)
© Dwight Eschliman: pages 163, 164, 167
© Darryl Estrine: pages iii, iv (shoulder detail), 43, 48-49, 66, 69, 74, 92, 94, 100 (man), 101, 106 (man), 108, 109 (man), 114, 119 (man), 121, 122 (man), 128, 133 (man), 134, 137 (man), 142, 143 (man)
© Dennis Galante: pages 12, 16
© Serge Krouglikoff/Image Bank/Getty Images: page 149 (left)
© Brian Bailey/Stone/Getty Images: page 156
© Philip North-Coombes/Stone/Getty Images: page 62
© LifeStock/Taxi/Getty Images: page 209
© John Hamel: page 186 (volleyball player)

© Mark Havriliak: page 78
© Donald Kinsella: page 166
© Image Library: page 159 (snake)
© Steven Lippman: page 54
© John Manno: pages 7, 9, 10, 18, 21, 22, 23
© Scott Markewitz: page 190
© Chris Milliman: page 206
© Todd Norwood: page 181
© PhotoDisc: pages 103, 149 (top right)
© Kate Powers: pages 24, 26
© Profimedia: page 88
© Tom Rafalovich: pages iv (runner), vi, 2, 150, 152
© Rodale Images: pages 62, 90, 217
© John Hamel/Rodale Images: pages 174, 185 (tennis), 189, 213, 215, 219 (baseball)
© Ed Landrock/Rodale Images: page 56, 91 (top), 210
© Mitch Mandel/Rodale Images: pages 29, 46, 159 (rabbit), 184
© Margaret Skrovanek/Rodale Images: page 34
© Charlie Samuels: page 195
© Gregg Segal: pages 160-161
© Piotr Sikora: pages 32, 36-37
© Stockbyte: pages 5, 86, 89, 175 (right)
© David Zickl: pages 180, 182, 183 (exercises), 185 (exercises), 186 (exercises), 187 (exercises)

Interior Illustrations
© Shawn Banner: pages 212, 213
© Molly Borman: pages iv (muscles), 100 (muscles), 106 (muscles), 109 (muscles), 119 (muscles), 122 (muscles), 133 (muscles), 137 (muscles), 143 (muscles)
© Julie Castillo: page 192 (tennis)
© Colin Hayes: pages 197, 198, 199, 200, 201, 202, 203
© Trevor Johnston: pages 192 (basketball), 193
© Zohar Lazar: pages 162, 165, 168
© Rod Little: page 195
© Ross MacDonald: page 170
© Mark Matcho: pages 28, 33, 63

Index

lat pulldown, 81, **81**
squat, 79–80, **80**
dangers of, 78–79
Cheddar cheese, 22
Cheese, 22
Cheesecake, 23
Chicken
baking, 13–16
crusted, 15–16
grilling, 16–17
marinades, 17
rubbed, 14
salmon compared to, 22–23
sauced, 14
stir-frying, 13
stuffed, 16
Chips, 21
Chromium, 29
Clock lunge, 155, **155**
Closed chain exercises, 71
Close-grip bench press, 112,
112
Cobbler's pose, 165
Cobra (warmup exercise), 68,
68
Cold showers, 63, 162
Coleslaw, 20
Complex carbohydrates, 4
Compound exercises
benefits of, 49
in workouts, 112
Concentration curl, 105, **105**
Cone slalom, 40–41
Conjugated linoleic acid, 17
Cooling
after workout, 63
during workout with fans, 59
Cooling vest, 166
Copperhead, 159
Core strength, cross-training
for, 168–69
Corn syrup, high-fructose, 29
Cravings, food, 5
Cross-knee twisting crunch, 53,
53

Cross-training, for
agility, 168
balance, 162–63
core strength, 168–69
endurance, 161–62
flexibility, 164–65
mental strength, 167–68
power/explosiveness, 163–64
runners, 153–54
time management, 166–67
upper-body strength, 165–66
Crunch, 95–96
Curb jump, 169

D

Dairy Ease, 28
Dance, 198
Deadlift, 48, 49–50
Romanian, 187, **187**
stiff-legged, 131
stiff-legged dumbbell, **144**,
144–45
Deltoids
benefits of strong, 115
exercises for
Arnold press, 116, **116**
barbell front raise, 117, **117**
barbell military press,
115–16
cable front raise, **117**,
117–18
cable two-arm raise, **118**,
118–19
dumbbell bent-over raise,
119, 119–20
dumbbell press, 116, **116**
lying incline-bench raise,
120, **120**
one-arm side raise, 118,
118
reverse pushup with
elbows out, 82
standing behind-the-neck
press, 116, **116**
Swiss-ball press, 116, **116**

muscle anatomy, 119, 119
workout for, 117, 118
Desserts, 23
DHT, 89
Diagonal chop, 36
Diet
meal-replacement shakes,
24–27
meals
breakfast, 8, 19–20
dinner, 11, 22–23
evening snack, 11
frequency, 7–11
lunch, 10, 20–21
midafternoon snack, 10–11
midmorning snack, 9–10
pitfalls
complacency, 5
food cravings, 5
hunger, 3
lack of results, 4
mood, 3–4
plateaus, 5–6
prescription drugs, 4
temptation, 6
weight gain, 90
yo-yo, 6
Dihydrotestosterone (DHT), 89
Dinner, 11, 22–23
Dog walking, 28
Donkey (warmup exercise), 68,
68
Double Swiss-ball pushup, **91**,
91
Downward dog, 165
Drop lunge, 186, **186**
Dry-land swimming, 147, **147**
Dumbbell alternating bench
press, 89
Dumbbell bench press, 52, **52**
Dumbbell bent-over raise, **119**,
119–20
Dumbbell curl, 105, **105**
Dumbbell hammer curl, 105,
105

S

Safety
  form shortcuts and, 78–79
  while trail-running, 158–59
Salad, 22
Salmon, 22–23
Salsa, 21
Sausage, 19
Scan Diet, 26
Scorpion (warmup exercise), 67,
    67
Scrambled eggs, 20
Seated calf raise, 127, **127**
Seated medicine-ball rotation,
    76, **76**
Seated medicine-ball throw, 75,
    75
Seated row, **142**, 142–44
Semimembranosus, **133**, 133
Semitendinosus, **133**, 133
Serotonin, 4
Sex, benefits of strong
  biceps, 102
  hamstrings, 128
  quadriceps and hip flexors,
    122–23
Shakes
  meal-replacement, 24–27
  milk in, 28
Shoulders
  benefits of strong, 115
  exercises for
    Arnold press, 116, **116**
    barbell front raise, 117,
      117
    barbell military press,
      115–16
    cable front raise, **117**,
      117–18
    cable two-arm raise, **118**,
      118–19
    dumbbell bent-over raise,
      119, 119–20
    dumbbell press, 116, **116**
    empty can, 166

lying incline-bench raise,
    120, **120**
  one-arm side raise, 118,
    118
  standing behind-the-neck
    press, 116, **116**
  Swiss-ball press, 116, **116**
muscle anatomy, **119**, 119
training with chest muscles,
    114–15
workout for, 117, 118
Shredder, **198**, 198–99
Shuttle run, 34
Side shuffle, 41
Single-arm cable row, **145**, 145
Single-arm extension, 113, **113**
Single-arm
    pulldown/pushdown,
    111, 111
Single-leg reach dips, 202, **202**
Single-leg sport-cord pullback,
    202, **202**
Single-leg squats on a foam ball,
    201, **201**
Single-leg standing reach-
    downs, 201, **201**
Sit and reach, 34
Situp, 33
Skater jump, 42
Skiing
  cross-country, 201–2, **202**
  dance training for, 198
  exercises for, 198–99,
    198–99
  moguls, 190, **190**
Slim-Fast, 25–27, 26
Snack
  choice
    candy vs. pretzel, 29
    popcorn vs. nachos, 21
    salsa vs. guacamole, 21
    Swiss vs. cheddar, 22
  evening, 11
  midafternoon, 10–11
  midmorning, 9–10

Snowboarding
  catching big air, **190**, 190–91
  exercises for, 200–201, **201**
Snowshoeing, 197–98, **198**
Soccer
  cross-training, 168
  injury prevention, 214, 214
Sore muscles, 41, 63, 71–72, 85,
    155, 162
Speed, breakaway, 182–83,
    183
Speed bench press, 165–66
Speed carioca, 41
Speed of lifting
  myths about, 70
  tempo of sets, 88
Speed rotation, 181
Speed skating, **199**, 199–200
Spice mixtures, 14
Split jumps, 180, **180**
Split squat, 149
Sports drinks, 155, 175
Spotter, 62
Squat
  barbell, 52, **52**
  dumbbell, **123**, 123
  fitness test, 33
  form, 79–80, 80, 123–25
  front, 123
  king, 82
  knee safety and, 71
  one-legged wall, 123
  single-leg on a foam ball, 201,
    201
  split, 149
  sumo, **123**, 123
Squat jump, 186
Squat-jump throw, 42
Squat to press, 187
Stability, strong quadriceps for,
    123
Staggered-stance dumbbell row,
    37
Stairclimber, 57
Stance, changing, 86